AF774089

Essentials in Ophthalmology

Series Editor

Arun D. Singh, Cleveland Clinic Foundation
Cole Eye Institute
Cleveland, OH, USA

Essentials in Ophthalmology aims to promote the rapid and efficient transfer of medical research into clinical practice. It is published in four volumes per year. Covering new developments and innovations in all fields of clinical ophthalmology, it provides the clinician with a review and summary of recent research and its implications for clinical practice. Each volume is focused on a clinically relevant topic and explains how research results impact diagnostics, treatment options and procedures as well as patient management.
The reader-friendly volumes are highly structured with core messages, summaries, tables, diagrams and illustrations and are written by internationally well-known experts in the field. A volume editor supervises the authors in his/her field of expertise in order to ensure that each volume provides cutting-edge information most relevant and useful for clinical ophthalmologists. Contributions to the series are peer reviewed by an editorial board.

Careen Y. Lowder
Nabin Shrestha • Arthi Venkat
Editors

Emerging Ocular Infections

Springer

Editors
Careen Y. Lowder
Department of Ophthalmology - Uveitis
Cleveland Clinic - Cole Eye Institute
Cleveland, OH, USA

Nabin Shrestha
Department of Infectious Diseases
Cleveland Clinic Foundation
Cleveland, USA

Arthi Venkat
Department of Ophthalmology -
Medical Retina and Uveitis
University of Virginia
Charlottesville, VA, USA

ISSN 1612-3212 ISSN 2196-890X (electronic)
Essentials in Ophthalmology
ISBN 978-3-031-24558-9 ISBN 978-3-031-24559-6 (eBook)
https://doi.org/10.1007/978-3-031-24559-6

© Springer Nature Switzerland AG 2023
This work is subject to copyright. All rights are reserved by the Publisher, whether the whole or part of the material is concerned, specifically the rights of translation, reprinting, reuse of illustrations, recitation, broadcasting, reproduction on microfilms or in any other physical way, and transmission or information storage and retrieval, electronic adaptation, computer software, or by similar or dissimilar methodology now known or hereafter developed.
The use of general descriptive names, registered names, trademarks, service marks, etc. in this publication does not imply, even in the absence of a specific statement, that such names are exempt from the relevant protective laws and regulations and therefore free for general use.
The publisher, the authors, and the editors are safe to assume that the advice and information in this book are believed to be true and accurate at the date of publication. Neither the publisher nor the authors or the editors give a warranty, expressed or implied, with respect to the material contained herein or for any errors or omissions that may have been made. The publisher remains neutral with regard to jurisdictional claims in published maps and institutional affiliations.

This Springer imprint is published by the registered company Springer Nature Switzerland AG
The registered company address is: Gewerbestrasse 11, 6330 Cham, Switzerland

Preface

The ability of infectious diseases to directly infect or incite secondary inflammatory responses in the eye brings to light an important connection between the specialties of Infectious Disease and Ophthalmology. Awareness of ocular manifestations of infectious diseases is crucially important for both ophthalmologists and infectious disease specialists alike.

Infectious agents that affect the eye come from all classes of microorganisms including viruses, bacteria, fungi, and parasites. These pathogens can affect multiple sites in the eye. Ocular manifestations of HIV, syphilis, tuberculosis, and members of the Herpesviridae family have been well recognized for decades. Infection may be limited to the eye, or eye involvement may be part of a multi-system infection. The anatomy of the eye and pharmacokinetic properties of antimicrobial agents in the eye require special considerations in administration of these medications. It may also be necessary to consider treatment of the infection outside the eye. Combined expertise of ophthalmology and infectious diseases maximizes the ability to make accurate diagnoses and provide appropriate management in infections that affect the eye.

Ocular manifestations of infectious diseases have continued to play an important role from a public health perspective in the last decade. A worldwide outbreak of cardiovascular infection caused by *Mycobacterium chimaera* associated with airborne contamination of heater-cooler units used in cardiovascular surgery, first reported in 2011, has prominent ophthalmological manifestations that can point to the diagnosis. A wide range of ocular manifestations have been reported during outbreaks such as the Ebola outbreak in West Africa between 2014 and 2016, and the COVID-19 pandemic in 2020.

In recent years, there have been major advancements in eye imaging technology, microbiological techniques (PCR, nucleic acid sequencing), and antimicrobial treatments (newer antimicrobials, ability to administer IV antimicrobials in patients' homes). These advances have occurred in multiple fields, making it difficult to keep pace. Collaboration between specialties provides an opportunity for these advances to be shared and utilized to improve our ability to diagnose and manage these complex conditions.

As the ocular and extra-ocular manifestations of infections can present diagnostic challenges, it is crucial that infectious disease specialists and ophthalmologists work together, embracing an interdisciplinary approach to diagnosis and management. This series is focused on emerging infections with eye manifestations being increasingly recognized or re-emerging older infections with important eye manifestations, with the various chapters organized by pathogen type.

It is our hope that this text can better inform the diagnostic and treatment decisions of both ophthalmologists and infectious disease specialists alike as we handle these complex diseases together.

Cleveland, OH, USA Careen Y. Lowder
Cleveland, USA Nabin Shrestha
Charlottesville, VA, USA Arthi Venkat

Contents

Ocular Tuberculosis

1

Aniruddha Agarwal, Vishali Gupta, and Lulette Tricia Bravo

Abbreviations

anti-VEGF	anti-vascular endothelial growth factor
ATT	anti-tuberculosis treatment
FAF	fundus autofluorescence
FFA	fundus fluorescein angiography
ICGA	indocyanine green angiography
IGRA	interferon-gamma release assay
IOTB	intraocular TB
OCT	optical coherence tomography
OCTA	OCT angiography
PCR	polymerase chain reaction
RPE	retinal pigment epithelium
TAU	TB-associated uveitis
TAU	tubercular anterior uveitis
TB	tuberculosis
TB SLC	tubercular serpiginous-like choroiditis
TBP	TB panuveitis
TBU	tuberculous uveitis
TIU	tubercular intermediate uveitis
TPU	tubercular posterior uveitis
TRV	TB retinal vasculitis
TST	tuberculin skin test
UWF	ultra-wide field

A. Agarwal · V. Gupta (✉)
Advanced Eye Centre, Postgraduate Institute of Medical Education and Research, Chandigarh, India

L. T. Bravo
Department of Infectious Disease, Cleveland Clinic, Cleveland, OH, USA
e-mail: bravot@ccf.org

Introduction

Mycobacterium tuberculosis affects a third of the world's population, with a reported 8.7 M new cases each year and approximately 1.4 M deaths annually [1, 2]. It is estimated that only 10 percent of infected people manifest with symptoms, mostly involving the lungs and the respiratory tract. In 2017, only 14% of symptomatic tuberculosis cases were reported to be extrapulmonary. The worldwide incidence of intraocular tuberculosis is variable and has shown a wide range in the literature—from 1.4% to 18% [3–7].

Tuberculosis (TB) is an airborne infection caused by *Mycobacterium tuberculosis.* It is much more common in the developing world and is associated with severe morbidity and mortality. Intraocular TB (IOTB) is a rare condition that often presents without clinical evidence of active pulmonary TB and may be the first and only manifestation of the infection [1, 8].

Posterior uveitis is the most common form of ocular TB, and early recognition with initiation of specific therapy is of paramount importance especially to prevent its visually debilitating manifestations [1, 9]. Patients with posterior uve-

© Springer Nature Switzerland AG 2023
C. Y. Lowder et al. (eds.), *Emerging Ocular Infections*, Essentials in Ophthalmology,
https://doi.org/10.1007/978-3-031-24559-6_1

itis due to TB represent the most challenging entities to diagnose and manage due to the diagnostic conundrums and similarity with other uveitic entities. Therefore, these cases are often misdiagnosed and incorrectly treated [10, 11].

IOTB can affect various ocular structures resulting in a wide spectrum of clinical manifestations. Some of these may be due to direct mycobacterial invasion of the ocular tissue, while others may be due to delayed hypersensitivity reaction to the bacteria. The disease may manifest with a variety of clinical signs and symptoms causing visual loss due to multiple reasons. Tuberculous uveitis (TBU) may present as anterior, intermediate, posterior, or panuveitis and can mimic various other infective as well as non-infective diseases [1, 9, 11, 12].

Establishing the diagnosis of IOTB is especially a challenge due to several reasons: (1) the disease can affect all ocular structures causing protean clinical manifestations; (2) gold standard tests like smear and/or culture positivity from ocular fluids have a poor yield owing to the difficulties in obtaining ocular samples combined with paucibacillary nature of the disease; and (3) high prevalence of TB in endemic countries makes it difficult to differentiate between true TBU and uveitis associated with unrelated latent TB [8, 11]. Thus, in real-world clinical practice, the phenotype recognition is a very important component of suspecting IOTB combined with corroborative evidence to make the diagnosis and initiate anti-TB therapy [9, 10]. Also it is very important to rule out other possible infections that might be prevalent in that geographic region.

Pathogenesis

M. tuberculosis is an aerobic acid-fast bacillus that has a high amount of lipid content in its cell wall. Humans are its only host and reservoir. As *M. tuberculosis* organisms are acquired via the inhalation route, they are engulfed by alveolar macrophages and dendritic cells. The organisms are then transported to the hilar lymph nodes and potentially to other distant extrapulmonary sites. This process is followed by increased cytokine production particularly IL-12 and TNF- alpha which in turn activate the TH1 cell-dominant adaptive immune response. The CD4 TH1 cell consequently produces IFN-gamma and TNF-alpha, which are crucial in the development of the cell-mediated immune response to *M. tuberculosis* and to granuloma formation [13]. Specific antigens like the early secretory antigenic target (ESAT-6) and culture filtrate protein (CFP-10) found in patients with TB can elicit vigorous helper T-cell responses causing cell lysis and subsequent bacterial dissemination [14, 15].

Pathogenesis of Intraocular Tuberculosis

There are several mechanisms through which *M. tuberculosis* can infect the eye. Most commonly, it can spread via the hematogenous route—it disseminates via the bloodstream to the eye from a remote primary source of infection [7]. In this pathway, the ciliary body and the choroid are the most frequently involved structures given their high vascular content and increased regional oxygen tension [16]. The retinal pigment epithelium (RPE) cells express Toll-like receptors which may actively phagocytose *M. tuberculosis* that reaches the inner choroid via the hematogenous route [17]. Once the intracellular *M. tuberculosis* reaches a sufficient number, a cytotoxic cell-mediated response leads to destruction of the macrophages and surrounding tissue and the formation of caseation [17].

Another process of ocular infection develops through primary exogenous infection of the eye. This is when *M. tuberculosis* directly infects the eyelids and the conjunctiva. Alternatively, a secondary infection can occur via direct extension from the eye's contiguous structures. For example, orbital TB (which is a rare form of ocular TB) is believed to be spread via the paranasal sinuses, presenting as periostitis, orbital soft tissue tuberculoma, or cold abscesses [18].

Finally, tuberculosis of the eye can present as an immune-mediated or hypersensitivity reaction to circulating *M. tuberculosis* antigens. In this mechanism, there is an inflammatory response to either an active tuberculosis infection outside the eye or to a latent infection. Phlyctenular keratoconjunctivitis, for instance, is a form of conjunctivitis derived from a delayed hypersensitivity response in the cornea or conjunctiva secondary to various pathogens such as *M. tuberculosis*, *Staphylococcus* species, and certain parasites [19, 20]. It presents as a nodule at the limbus or on the conjunctiva.

Overall, among these proposed mechanisms of disease, the precise events leading to tuberculous uveitis and intraocular tuberculosis remain unclear and continue to be controversial [21]. There is no experimental model that can explain all the clinical manifestations of TBU, and thus it is quite likely that different mechanisms may be playing role to produce different manifestations.

Clinical Features

Clinical manifestations of IOTB are variable, which pose a challenge for diagnosis. The commonest form of reported uveitis in TB is tubercular posterior uveitis (TPU) followed by tubercular panuveitis (TBP), tubercular intermediate uveitis (TIU), and tubercular anterior uveitis (TAU) [1, 8–10, 22]. Tuberculosis can potentially involve any part of the eye, and thus, there is no single pathognomonic presentation. Aside from tuberculosis, there are other etiologies for granulomatous inflammation of the eye which may present with similar ophthalmologic findings and may thus, at times, cause diagnostic uncertainty. Differential diagnoses include sarcoidosis, syphilis, sympathetic ophthalmia, uveitis associated with multiple sclerosis, lens-induced uveitis intraocular foreign body, Vogt-Koyanagi-Harada syndrome, and other infectious etiologies [23].

The incidence of ocular involvement in patients with pulmonary TB is variable ranging from 1.4% to, more recently, 6.8%, in a later study [4, 24, 25]. Its incidence rate may vary with location. It has been reported to be 0.3% in South India [26], while it is 11.7% in North India [27].

Among HIV-positive patients, choroidal granuloma has been the most common presentation described in studies [28]. In a retrospective case series of patients coinfected with HIV and tuberculosis in South India, 15 out of 766 patients were diagnosed to have ocular TB. These patients presented with choroidal granuloma (52%), subretinal abscess (37%) some of which worsened to panophthalmitis, and lastly a case each of conjunctival tuberculosis (5.2%) and panophthalmitis (5.2%). All these patients had concomitant pulmonary tuberculosis, and CD4 counts ranged from 14 to 560 cells/μL (mean 160). Severity and incidence of ocular manifestations were not found to correlate with CD4 counts. The relatively higher number of panophthalmitis cases were attributed to presence of impaired cell-mediated immunity in this population of patients. One case of panophthalmitis had happened after a robust rise in CD4 cell counts following antiretroviral treatment and was felt to be from paradoxical worsening or immune reconstitution inflammatory syndrome (IRIS) [28].

A higher incidence of ocular involvement (18%) was noted among 100 patients with tuberculosis admitted to a general hospital in a prospective study of microbiologically confirmed tuberculosis cases done in the AIDS era [5]. The study group included both HIV-positive and HIV-negative patients. Like the prior study, the authors similarly did not detect a significant difference in CD4 counts among HIV-infected patients who had ocular tuberculosis versus those who did not. All 18 patients with ocular tuberculosis had concomitant systemic tuberculosis, with 11 not reporting any ocular symptoms. Multivariable analysis showed that miliary disease (odds ratio 43.92, $p = 0.002$), ocular symptoms (odds ratio 6.35 and $p = 0.0143$), and decreased visual acuity (odds ratio (0.04, $p = 0.012$) were the independent risk factors that predicted for ocular involvement. Miliary disease was the most significant risk factor in both HIV-infected and HIV-negative groups. The presence of HIV infection by itself was not found to be statistically associated with ocular tuberculosis.

In TB-endemic areas, broad-based posterior synechiae, retinal vasculitis with or without choroiditis, and serpiginous-like choroiditis have been found to be highly specific for tubercular uveitis with a specificity, likelihood ratio, and posttest probability of 79%, 93%, and 90%, respectively [29]. Gupta et al., in their retrospective comparative case study, proposed that a patient with these clinical features should further undergo testing for active or latent tuberculosis by proceeding with tuberculin skin test, QuantiFERON-TB Gold test, or chest imaging in the form of chest x-ray or CT chest [30].

In non-endemic areas, however, the diagnosis of ocular tuberculosis may be more challenging and is typically made presumptively. There are no uveitis features that are pathognomonic, and various ocular features may range from nongranulomatous anterior uveitis to occlusive retinal vasculitis [31]. Radiographic studies do not typically show abnormalities or signs of pulmonary involvement. The main exam finding is a chronic resistant granulomatous uveitis [32]. Many times, the diagnosis is based presumptively on a positive QuantiFERON-TB Gold test and/or a tuberculin skin test, further confirmed retrospectively if resolution of the inflammation occurs with antituberculosis treatment.

Tubercular Anterior Uveitis (TAU)

TB anterior uveitis often presents as chronic granulomatous disease which may be unilateral or bilateral. It is characterized by large, mutton fat keratic precipitates, iris nodules which may be present near the pupillary border (Koeppe) or on the iris surface (Busacca), and broad-based posterior synechiae [8, 33]. The disease can be complicated by the development of cataract with or without accompanying vitritis. Broad-based posterior synechiae have been described as a hallmark sign of TAU, a sign that is predictive of possible tubercular etiology. Rarely, TB can also present as non-granulomatous uveitis including hypopyon [1, 8, 30, 33].

Tubercular Intermediate Uveitis (TIU)

The presentation of TIU is non-specific with a waxing and waning course. Patients generally present with smoldering, chronic uveitis characterized by the presence of vitritis, snowball opacities, and peripheral vascular sheathing and may in addition have retinochoroidal granulomas [10, 34–36]. The disease may be complicated by cystoid macular edema or cataract and less commonly by glaucoma/ocular hypertension, epiretinal membrane (ERM) formation, retinal detachment, peripheral neovascularization, or vitreous hemorrhage [1, 8].

Tubercular Posterior Uveitis (TPU) and TB Panuveitis (TBP)

Posterior uveitis is the most common ocular manifestation of IOTB and may be unilateral or bilateral. Choroid is the primary site of involvement with lesions varying from choroidal tubercles and choroidal granulomas to serpiginous-like choroiditis [8]. Retinitis as sole manifestation of TB is rare, and usually there is associated choroiditis. However, TB may present as retinal vasculitis that tends to be occlusive in nature [37, 38].

Choroidal Tubercles/Tuberculoma

Choroidal tubercles are one of the most characteristic intraocular manifestations of TB usually seen in disseminated disease. These tubercles have been defined as "single/multiple, small (≤ 0.5 disc diameter), discreet greyish-white lesions with a central core and surrounding rim of inflammation typically in a patient with miliary disease" [39]. They are small yellowish, discrete lesions generally smaller than a quarter disc diameter with ill-defined borders, located deep in the choroid (Fig. 1.1). Associated anterior segment or vitreous inflammation is usually not seen. When healed, these tubercles appear better circumscribed with surrounding pigment and may develop into a scar [8, 39–43].

Solitary Choroidal Tuberculoma/Subretinal Abscess

Untreated choroidal tubercles may grow in size up to 14 mm or more, to present as solitary elevated mass-like lesion known as choroidal tuberculoma. Choroidal tuberculomas have been defined as single/multiple yellowish subretinal

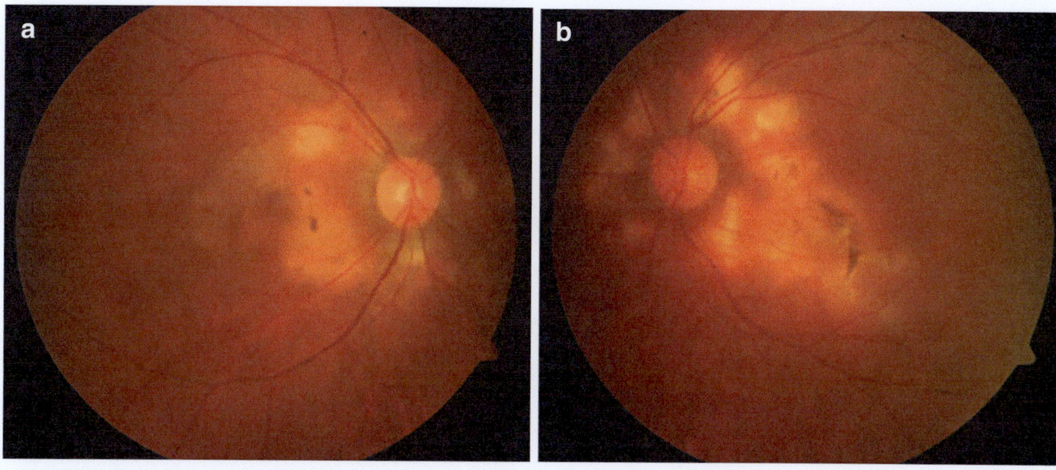

Fig. 1.1 Figure shows two patients with tubercular choroidal granulomas (tuberculomas). In patient 1 (**a**), the tuberculomas are multiple and present in the peripapillary region as yellow, raised, voluminous lesions with surrounding fluid and exudation. Similar lesions are observed in patient 2 (**b**), along with central scarring and pigmentation

lesion with indistinct borders and surrounding exudative fluid, along with oval/round lesion in the choroidal stroma. This would include tubercular subretinal abscess (severe form with exudation, rapid necrosis and tissue destruction, and overlying retinal hemorrhages) [22]. These tuberculomas may be mistaken for tumors, and eyes may be enucleated for mistaken diagnosis. There is underlying tissue destruction resulting from progressive, liquefied caseation necrosis with rapid multiplication of tubercular bacilli. They may even break into vitreous cavity and mimic subretinal abscess causing widespread intraocular inflammation [8, 44, 45].

Tubercular Serpiginous-Like Choroiditis (TB SLC)

TB SLC represents an immune-mediated hypersensitivity reaction to the acid-fast bacilli (*Mycobacterium tuberculosis*) sequestrated in the RPE. It is different from the classic autoimmune variety as it predominantly affects younger population with mostly bilateral lesions which are noncontiguous to optic disc. TB SLC have been defined as "single/multiple discreet yellowish-white fuzzy choroidal lesions and slightly raised edges that show wave-like progression with an active serpiginous-like edge with central healing" (Fig. 1.2). TB SLC lesions can further be *multifocal* or *placoid* [30, 46–49]. The patients with TB SLC can be differentiated from autoimmune variety of serpiginous choroiditis as eyes with TB SLC tend to show presence of vitritis, multifocality with skip lesions with or without peripheral vasculitis [30, 46].

Two different presentations of the disease are:

1. *Multifocal choroiditis*: In this phenotype of SLC, there are discrete lesions, yellowish-white in color with well-defined margins and slightly raised edges. The edges of these lesions are noncontiguous at first and progress relentlessly over a period of 1–4 weeks to a diffuse, contiguous variety, acquiring an active advancing edge [46].
2. *Plaque-like choroiditis*: This phenotype has solitary diffuse plaque-like lesion which shows amoeboid spread. These lesions have elevated active edges, while the center of the lesion heals with pigmentation [46].

TB Retinal Vasculitis (TRV)

TRV has been defined as isolated retinal vasculitis (either periphlebitis and/or arteritis) with/without occlusive disease [37, 38]. Vasculitis in patients with tuberculosis suggests an immune-mediated hypersensitivity response to the bacteria with phlebitis being an important clinical

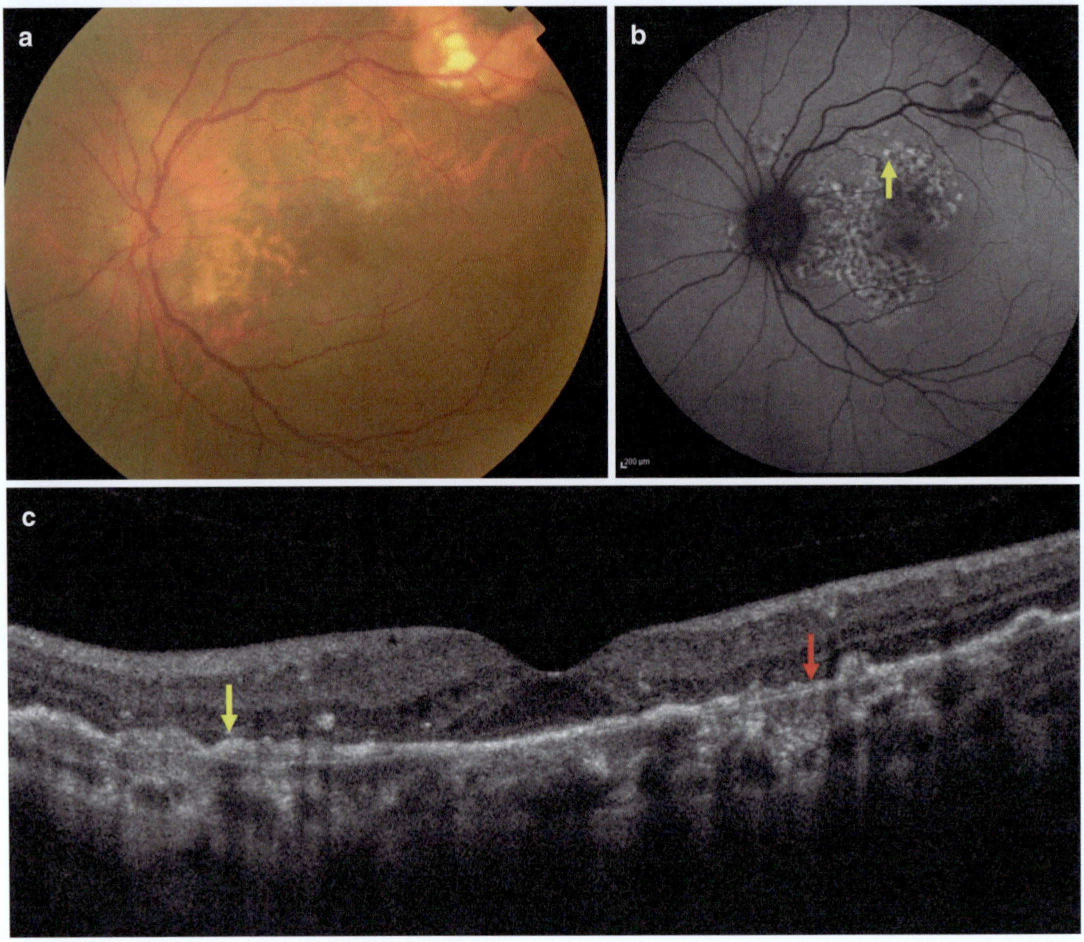

Fig. 1.2 (**a**) Fundus photography of a 28-year-old male with tubercular serpiginous-like choroiditis shows presence of yellowish-white choroiditis lesions at the posterior pole with fuzzy edges and ill-defined margins and pigmented choroidal lesions temporal to fovea. (**b**) Fundus autofluorescence (FAF) imaging of the same eye shows areas of speckled autofluorescence with hyperfluorescent edges (yellow arrow) corresponding to activity at the edges. Temporally lesions are hypo-autofluorescent (stage 4) suggestive of inactive lesions. (**c**) Swept-source OCT (SS-OCT) of the left eye passing through the fovea shows hyperreflectivity of outer retinal layers (yellow arrow) nasal to fovea. Corresponding to healed lesions, there is loss of RPE and outer retinal layers (red arrow) seen just temporal to fovea. As the edges are still active, there is a need for continued anti-tubercular therapy and systemic immunosuppression

finding. The predilection for retinal veins in tubercular retinal vasculitis and its clinical features resemble Eales' disease. Patients with active tubercular vasculitis demonstrate vitritis, neuroretinitis, perivascular cuffing by the exudates, retinal/vitreous hemorrhage, cystoid macular edema, occlusive features in the form of capillary non-perfusion of the retina, or neovascularization of the optic disc/retina [38, 50, 51]. Perivascular choroiditis lesions are quite specific indicators of TB etiology (see Fig. 1.2) [52]. The occlusive retinal vasculitis in TB tends to produce areas of capillary non-perfusion with development of neovascularization that may result in vitreous hemorrhages that may be mistaken as Eales' disease (Fig. 1.3) [53–55].

Endophthalmitis and Panophthalmitis

Rarely TB can present as acute-onset endogenous endophthalmitis with vitritis and hypopyon. It may occur due to rapid multiplication

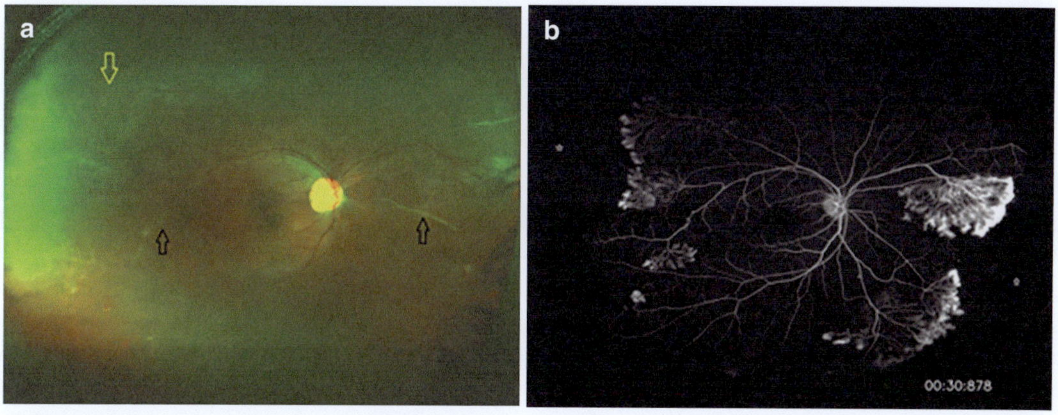

Fig. 1.3 A 30-year-old male with decreased vision in left eye for the past 1 month. Left eye had vitreous hemorrhage (not shown). (**a**) Ultrawide-field (UWF) fundus photography of the right eye showed mild vitritis with sheathing of vessels mainly veins (black arrows) and peripheral large neovascular tufts (yellow arrow). (**b**) UWF fluorescein angiography of the same eye in the late venous phase confirmed the presence of large neovascularization complexes both nasally and temporally with peripheral non-perfusion areas (white asterisk). The patient had a positive tuberculin skin test. He was started on oral corticosteroids and anti-tubercular therapy. Peripheral scatter laser of the non-perfused areas was performed

of acid-fast bacilli or in patients who receive corticosteroid therapy without concomitant antitubercular drugs [56, 57].

Tubercular Optic Neuropathy

Optic nerve involvement in TB may reflect direct infection induced by the mycobacteria or from a hypersensitivity to the infectious agent. It might manifest as neuroretinitis, papilledema, papillitis, optic neuritis, retrobulbar neuritis, or optic nerve tubercle. The neuroretinitis may result from contiguous spread of the organisms to the juxtapapillary retina from the choroid or from disseminated hematogenous spread of the TB organisms from the pulmonary or other primary infectious focus [58–60].

Tuberculosis of Ocular Adnexa

Mycobacteria rarely affect the scleral tissue leading to either diffuse or nodular TB scleritis. These cases are usually difficult to diagnose and need to be differentiated from autoimmune scleritis [61–63]. However, if left untreated, they may progress to cause scleral necrosis and perforation. Orbital TB may manifest as periostitis, dacryoadenitis, soft tissue tuberculoma, osteomyelitis, or a cold abscess. TB of conjunctiva is extremely rare; however, nodular inflammation phlyctenular keratoconjunctivitis may be a delayed hypersensitivity reaction to mycobacterial antigens [64].

Laboratory Testing

There has been no clear gold standard test for the diagnosis of ocular tuberculosis and thus no consensus regarding its diagnostic criteria. A definitive diagnosis would require isolation of *M. tuberculosis* in tissue or ocular fluid culture. However, due to the technical difficulty and risks of proceeding with obtaining ocular fluid, coupled with the paucibacillary nature of the disease associated with low sensitivity of culture and PCR testing, distinguishing between active TB of the eye and an immune-mediated reaction to a distant focus of infection or latent TB becomes challenging. This has led to significant heterogeneity in the approach to the diagnosis and management of intraocular tuberculosis among various referral centers in the world [65, 66].

Direct Laboratory Evidence of *M. tuberculosis* Ocular Infection

Mycobacterial culture is the gold standard for diagnosing *M. tuberculosis* infection. It allows for organism species and strain identification and susceptibility testing. On solid media, it takes 3–8 weeks for *M. tuberculosis* to grow, whereas on liquid media, growth is facilitated and can be detected within 7–21 days. Nucleic acid amplification can offer direct detection in clinical specimens and thus can provide the advantage of a more rapid diagnosis and turnaround time. Gene Xpert MTB/RIF assay is recommended by WHO for the rapid diagnosis of tuberculosis. It can detect both the presence of *M. tuberculosis* in clinical specimens and also rifampin resistance by determining the presence of rpoB gene mutations. The typical turnaround time is 2 h. Its use in diagnosing ocular tuberculosis is worth studying. In a recent study of 714 patients' samples (285 from pulmonary and 429 from extrapulmonary sources), the sensitivity and the specificity of GeneXpert MTB/RIF were almost similar in both groups (78.2% and 90.4%, and 79.3% and 90.3%, respectively) [67].

In ocular tuberculosis, confirming the diagnosis by identifying *M. tuberculosis* in an ocular specimen is usually very challenging given the relatively low sensitivity of these diagnostic tests, the paucibacillary nature of the disease, and the potential complications of the diagnostic procedure which include visual loss, retinal detachment, and infection [21]. In addition, it is uncommon to find histopathologic evidence of necrotizing granulomatous inflammation among clinical cases since this would need a fairly large ocular biopsy sample to establish a diagnosis [68, 69]. Overall, ocular TB diagnosis remains a clinical or presumptive diagnosis based on the summative results of the patient's history, physical exam findings, radiographic evidence, and other supporting lab results. Given this, there is a heterogenous approach to the diagnosis and management of ocular tuberculosis throughout the world, and no clear consensus has been reached [21].

Polymerase Chain Reaction

Polymerase chain reaction (PCR) from intraocular fluids for the diagnosis of TB has limited application in real-world scenario as only one-third of patients with suspected TBU may be positive for *Mycobacterium tuberculosis* on PCR [53, 70–72]. Moreover, there is lack of standardization of PCR. Factors affecting sensitivity and specificity include volume of sample, number of amplification targets, and DNA extraction method, with inhibitors in the fluid sample. Due to lack of sensitivity of current PCR techniques, a positive PCR may be considered reliable if the phenotype is suggestive of TB and other possible causes have been ruled out. However, negative results do not exclude TBU [72].

Ancillary Ocular Investigations

Color Photography and Ultra-Wide Field Imaging

Color fundus photography helps in accurately identifying the morphology of the IOTB lesions, and serial imaging at regular intervals aids in objective assessment of change in lesions over an extended period of time [73]. Ultra-wide field (UWF) fundus too is a useful adjunct to identify peripheral active TB vasculitis, peripheral neovascularization, and areas of non-perfusion requiring laser which might be missed on conventional imaging modalities [52].

Fundus Autofluorescence

Fundus autofluorescence (FAF) is a noninvasive imaging technique that details the health of the RPE. As RPE and choriocapillaris are the proposed major sites of involvement in TB SLC, FAF can play an important role in assessing disease activity and resolution of such lesions. Gupta et al. [74, 75] have described different stages in the resolution of SLC lesions using FAF imaging (see Fig. 1.2). The acute stage (stage 1) shows an ill-defined amorphous lesion with halo-like hyper-autofluorescence and ill-defined margins. As the lesion starts healing, a thin rim of hypo-autofluorescence is seen surrounding the lesion which remains predominantly hyper-autofluorescent with a stippled pattern (stage 2). With further healing, there is increasing hypo-autofluorescence in an outward-in fashion, and the lesion shows predominant hypo-autofluorescence (stage 3) on FAF imaging. The entire lesion becomes hypo-autofluorescent (stage 4) on complete resolution, and this marks the end of activity and RPE atrophy.

Fundus Fluorescein Angiography (FFA)

The active lesions in TB SLC appear hypofluorescent in the early phase and hyperfluorescent in the late phase (Fig. 1.4). Areas of resolution show

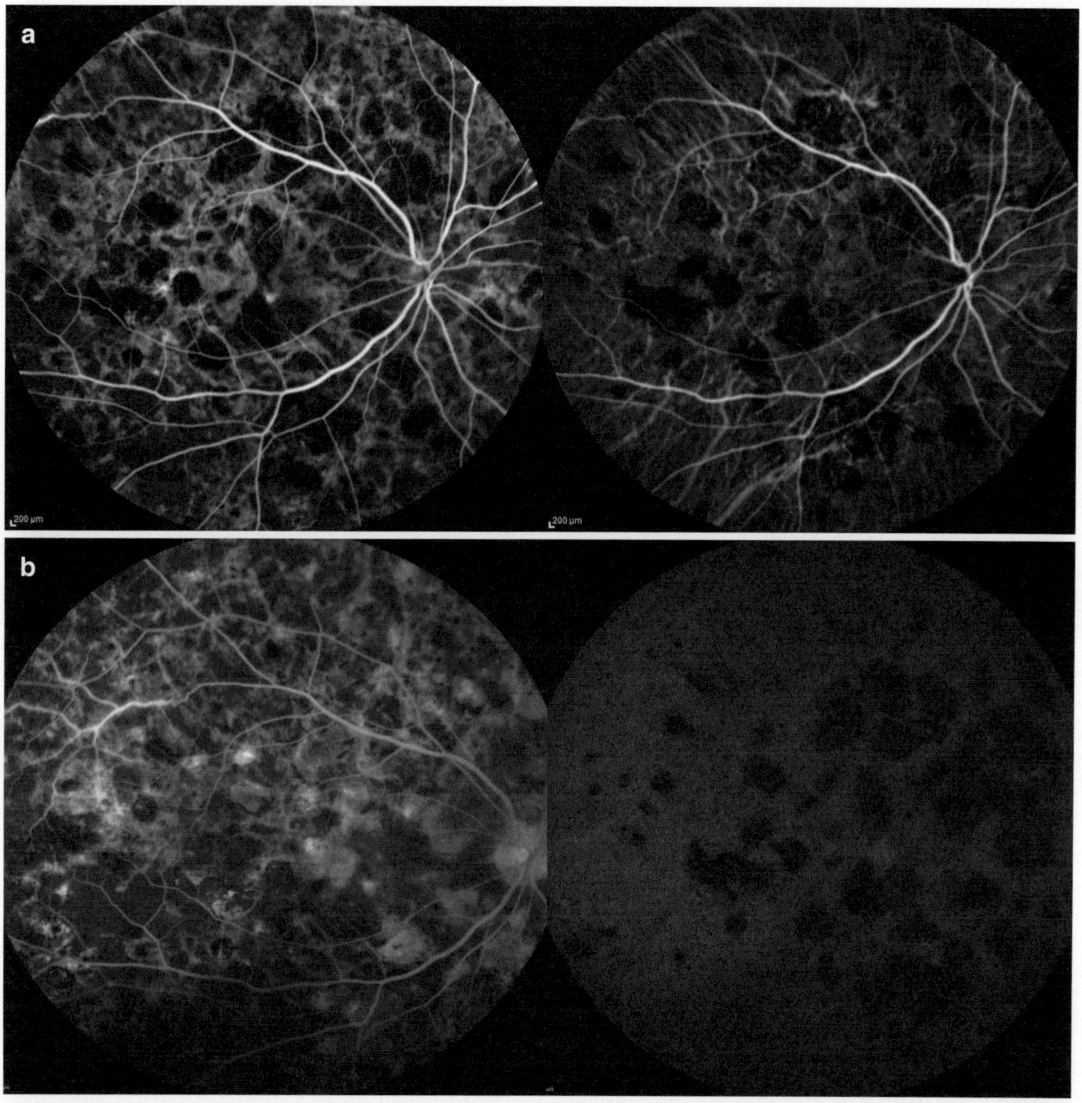

Fig. 1.4 Combined fluorescein angiography (FA) and indocyanine green angiography (ICGA) in the early (**a**) and late phase (**b**) in a young female with tubercular serpiginous-like choroiditis. The FA shows presence of early hypofluorescence and late hyperfluorescence with fuzziness of the active lesions, and transmission defects in the areas of choriocapillaris atrophy. ICGA imaging shows hypofluorescence in both early and late frames along with visible underlying choroidal vasculature in areas with choriocapillaris atrophy

transmission defects due to RPE damage and choriocapillaris atrophy. Also complications such as inflammatory choroidal neovascularization may be detected using FFA, though it may be very challenging in the absence of high index of suspicion [40, 76].

TB granulomas would also block choroidal fluorescence in the early phases as it does not have its own separate vascular supply. However, in the late phases, it may become intensely hyperfluorescent due to large amount of dye accumulating in the lesion. Being an inflammatory choroidal pathology, a TB choroidal granuloma may also be associated with an exudative detachment showing late phases pooling of the dye [8, 39, 40, 60]. Tuberculomas may sometimes be associated with deep retinal and subretinal hemorrhages in which case FFA helps in ruling out development of a secondary choroidal neovascularization or a retinal angiomatous proliferation-like lesion.

UWF FFA plays a significant role in identifying peripheral vascular leakage in cases of active TB vasculitis. Moreover since TB vasculitis is occlusive in nature, it can help identify neovascularization and areas of peripheral non-perfusion which would require scatter photocoagulation [52].

Indocyanine Green Angiography

Indocyanine green angiography (ICGA) is a useful tool in detecting choriocapillaritis and presence of choriocapillaris hypoperfusion among patients with IOTB (see Fig. 1.4). Active lesions of TB SLC remain hypofluorescence from early to late phase on ICGA. Two different ICG presentations are seen with TB choroidal granuloma based upon the thickness of the lesion in the choroidal stroma. Full-thickness choroidal involvement is seen as hypofluorescence in all phases of angiography, whereas partial choroidal thickness involvement is seen as early hypofluorescence becoming iso- or hyperfluorescent in mid and later phases [77]. Other changes of tubercular uveitis include fuzzy appearance of choroidal vessels in the intermediate phase and late choroidal hyperfluorescence due to dye leakage which tends to regress following therapy [1, 8, 40, 77].

Optical Coherence Tomography (OCT)

Acute SLC lesions correspond to outer retinal layer hyper-reflectivity on OCT with involvement of RPE, photoreceptor outer segment tips, ellipsoid region, ELM, and outer nuclear layer with a minimal involvement of inner retinal layers. With onset of resolution, the hyper-reflective regions are replaced by knobby irregular elevations of outer retinal layers. With further healing of lesions, a loss of outer retinal layers with increased choroidal backscattering has been reported (see Fig. 1.2) [40, 49, 74, 78, 79].

TB granulomas are seen as lobulated and nonhomogeneous on EDI-OCT. These granulomas may show increased transmission signal as compared to normal surrounding choroid. OCT can also help in differentiating choroidal tumors from inflammatory granulomas as the latter tend to have a smooth lesional surface and moderate thickness, unlike the often irregular topography and greatly increased choroidal thickness of choroidal tumors [40, 80, 81].

Recent introduction of OCT angiography (OCTA), a dye-less noninvasive technique, has furthered our capabilities to understand the pathological involvement in IOTB. OCTA was found to be effective in clearly delineating the lesion of CNV and detailing the involvement of retinochoroidal layers with branching vascular networks (Fig. 1.5) [49, 78, 82].

IFN-Gamma Release Assays (IGRA)

Other adjunctive tests include immunological tests such as the tuberculin skin test (TST) and interferon-gamma (IFN-gamma) release assay (IGRA) and chest imaging studies. The TST sensitivity for active TB is approximately 70% [83]. Its sensitivity and specificity for ocular TB range from 92% to 95% and 72% to 90%, respectively [84, 85]. False positives, however, may occur among populations that receive the BCG vaccine or those infected with certain nontuberculous mycobacterial infections that cross-react with the purified protein derivative used for the skin test.

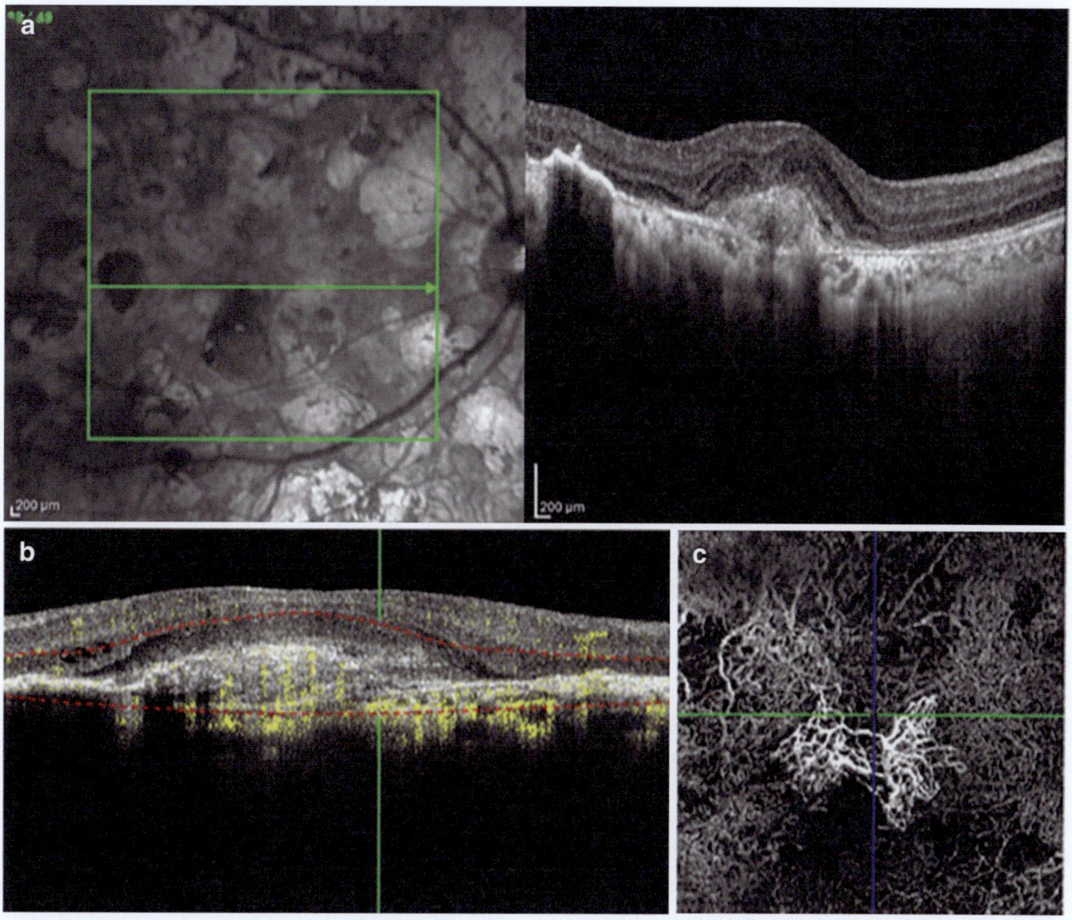

Fig. 1.5 Optical coherence tomography (OCT) and OCT angiography (OCTA) in a young male with healed tubercular serpiginous-like choroiditis. The OCT imaging shows presence of subretinal hyper-reflective material (SHRM) with streak of subretinal fluid indicating presence of choroidal neovascularization (**a**). The cross-sectional B-scan image obtained using OCTA confirms the presence of active CNV with flow signals (**b**). The en face OCTA scan shows an exuberant type 2 CNV (**c**)

Specificity for diagnosing tuberculosis infection is increased through the use of IGRAs: QuantiFERON TB-Gold (QFN-TB) and T-SPOT-TB. QFN-TB measures the amount of IFN-gamma produced by an individual's T cells when incubated for 24 hours with specific *M. tuberculosis* antigens such as ESAT6 and CFP10. The IFN gamma concentration is determined using optical density. T-SPOT-TB determines the amount of peripheral blood T cells secreting IFN-gamma represented by the number of spot footprints using the ELISpot technique. The antigens used by IGRA are specific to *M. tuberculosis* (ESAT6, CFP10, and TB7.7), and specificity in populations at low risk for latent TB infection ranges from 92% to 97% [83]. Sensitivity of IGRAs is fairly similar to TST for diagnosing active TB (76%) and latent TB. In a retrospective review of 82 cases of presumed ocular TB which described anti-tuberculosis treatment (ATT) response and association with QFN-TB, steroid use did not have a significant association with QFN-TB values and did not appear to affect QFT-TB accuracy [85].

Although IGRA is recognized to have a higher specificity than TST for the diagnosis of active or latent tuberculosis, there are also certain pitfalls with its use. Its positive predictive value is lower in populations that have a lower pretest probability [86, 87]. Some studies propose a higher cutoff value to increase the likelihood of a positive response to ATT [88].

It is important to consider other potential etiologies for uveitis and exclude these prior to making a diagnosis of ocular tuberculosis, even among those who have a positive IGRA result. The differential diagnoses include sarcoidosis, Behcet's, syphilis, and toxoplasmosis. For instance, in one study 25% of patients with uveitis and a positive QuantiFERON were found to have other causes [89]. Another study showed 37 out of 80 were found to have an alternative etiology, most cases secondary to intraocular sarcoidosis. IGRA should be checked selectively and only in those individuals who have a good pretest probability of TB infection such as those with a history of TB exposures or those with an idiopathic chronic inflammation that have had a suboptimal response to immunosuppression [9].

In a prospective cohort study of patients with clinical ocular signs of TB-associated uveitis (TAU), TST (72%) was found to be more sensitive than TSpot (36%), but TSpot (75%) was more specific than TST (51%). It was found however that if patients were positive for both TST and TSpot, they were 2.16 times more likely to have TAU. The authors thus recommended using both tests in addition to the presence of clinical ocular signs in diagnosing TB uveitis [90].

Chest Imaging

Most patients with tuberculous uveitis do not have associated extraocular manifestations. Majority of the time, especially in non-endemic regions, chest imaging is negative for signs of tuberculous involvement.

In a study of patients presenting with uveitis of unknown cause in South Africa, CXRs were normal/indeterminate in 88 out of 104 patients. Abnormal CXRs were present in 5 of 34 cases of IOTB (14.7%) versus 62.5% (5 of 8 cases) of intraocular sarcoidosis (IOS). CXR had a sensitivity of 14.7% and a specificity of 94.3% for intraocular TB compared with a sensitivity of 62.5% and specificity of 96.9% for IOS. The overall diagnostic accuracy of CXR was only 54.5% for IOTB, whereas it was higher at 79.9% for IOS [91].

Treatment of Intraocular Tuberculosis

There is little evidence available in the literature to help guide the management of ocular tuberculosis. Majority of studies are retrospective, and there are no randomized controlled trials to compare treatment outcomes. Thus, various referral centers in the world have attempted at least to develop a pathway or standardization of care for individuals who present with uveitis of unknown etiology that have had a suboptimal response to standard therapy [23, 92].

Several studies have described successful outcomes starting empiric ATT in presumed ocular tuberculosis [93–96]. In a retrospective study of 48 patients in the UK with presumed TB uveitis and positive IGRA, 6 months of ATT was given with complete resolution in 60% [93]. In a tertiary uveitis clinic in New Zealand, 30 patients with presumed TB uveitis were treated with 6–12 months of ATT, and 67% went into remission for at least 12 months [95]. Disappearance of ocular inflammation and response to ATT have likewise been reported in 60–70% of patients after ATT [31, 88]. A prospective case study of 96 patients presenting with ocular inflammation to an ophthalmology clinic in France described the outcome of 25 patients with positive QuantiFERON-TB Gold who were treated with 6 months ATT (6 of 25 with accompanying systemic steroids). The median QuantiFERON-TB Gold value was significantly higher in the patient group with a successful treatment response (7.67 IU/mL [0.46 to 33.37]) versus the group that did not improve (1.22 IU/mL [0.61 to 4.4]). The authors suggested considering a higher cutoff QuantiFERON-TB Gold value (>2 IU/mL) in helping identify patients who would more likely benefit from ATT [88].

Management of Intraocular Inflammation

The goal of therapy in TBU is to control current episode of inflammation to prevent any damage to intraocular structures and to prevent recurrences over a long-term follow-up. Intraocular inflammation is mainly controlled by the use of corticosteroids [46]. Systemic immunosuppressive agents may be considered when inflammation is not controlled by steroids. However, systemic corticosteroid or other immunosuppressive therapy should not be prescribed alone, and specific therapy in the form of ATT needs to be added for two reasons: (1) addition of ATT has shown to reduce recurrences over long-term follow-up by more than 80% [90, 97]. A report by the Collaborative Ocular TB Study (COTS) group on long-term follow-up of more than 24 months of treatment with ATT indicated that more than 75% of these patients are able to achieve cure [98]. (2) Treatment with systemic corticosteroids and immunosuppressive therapy in patients with latent TB may cause a flare-up of systemic TB by activating a latent infection [10, 48, 73, 97].

Tuberculosis screening should be performed ideally before immunosuppression is started among those patients who have had uveitis of unknown etiology that have not responded to conventional treatment and those with ocular findings suggestive of ocular tuberculosis [23]. Evaluation includes a combination of obtaining a clinical history, chest imaging, immunological testing, and sputum collection (if indicated) and, if feasible, obtaining an ocular specimen for mycobacterial culture or acid-fast bacilli PCR. HIV screening should be performed in all patients with presumed ocular TB. If workup is not definitive for a diagnosis of ocular tuberculosis but the clinical features point to active TB, a presumptive diagnosis can be made and initiation of an anti-tuberculosis regimen considered. Among clinical features, choroidal granulomas, occlusive retinal vasculitis, and multifocal serpiginoid choroiditis have been found to be most strongly predictive of ocular TB [99, 100]. Among these in particular, choroidal granulomas should raise a high index of suspicion especially since the inability to recognize it could lead to severe complications [101]. Lastly, ophthalmologists should also consider involving infectious disease in evaluating patients who continue to have a nondiagnostic workup. Reviewing with an infectious disease consultant the need for further CT chest imaging or PET scan may be of benefit in some situations [102].

The major challenge, however, in possible tubercular uveitis is defining the indications for initiating ATT as this decision is based on institutional and country practices and very often requires involvement of infectious disease specialists who may not be convinced to initiate ATT only for ocular disease in the absence of any direct evidence of infection. The COTS Consensus group tried to define the indications of initiating ATT. The experts took into consideration the phenotype, endemicity, immunological tests (TST skin test and QuantiFERON TB Gold ®), and radiologic evidence that mostly shows evidence of past exposure to TB in the form of calcified hilar nodes and not active disease. There was consensus to treat any form of TB choroiditis if any one of immunological and one radiologic test was positive. For phenotypes like TB SLC and tuberculomas, even one immunologic test alone without any radiologic evidence was considered sufficient for initiating ATT [103]. However, for phenotypes like TAU, the experts felt the need to treat only if disease was recurrent. Experts agreed on initiating ATT in TIU and active TRV only when one immunologic along with radiologic test was positive [104].

Anti-tuberculosis Treatment

ATT for ocular tuberculosis is similar to the treatment regimen for pulmonary tuberculosis, i.e., four drugs consisting of rifampin, isoniazid, pyrazinamide, and ethambutol for 8 weeks followed by isoniazid and rifampin for 4–10 months [103–105]. Some experts recommend co-management with infectious disease for assistance with antibiotic treatment and addressing potential side effects [21]. Ethambutol can lead to optic neuropathy, and monitoring for toxicity at follow-up every 2 months is recommended [23]. Ethambutol should be discontinued as soon as signs of ocular signs or symptoms of optic neuropathy appear (decreased visual acuity or abnormal ocular testing). Moxifloxacin has been used as an alternative to ethambutol, but there are experts who feel that the risk for ethambutol toxicity is relatively low and does not justify modifying the standard treatment regimen [93].

The duration of antibiotic treatment ranges from 6 to 9 months. There is no consensus regarding the optimal duration of ATT although there are some who recommend at least 9 months of treatment or longer. A higher success rate was found among patients with presumed ocular TB who received ATT for 9 months or longer, whereas poorer outcomes were associated with those on immunosuppression [106]. In a case-control study done by Ang et al., an 11-fold reduction in the likelihood of recurrence was noted among those patients with uveitis and latent TB treated with >9 months of ATT [90].

Paradoxical Worsening of IOTB

Paradoxical worsening of the disease also known as ocular Jarisch-Herxheimer reaction is an entity described in a subset of patients with extrapulmonary TB. It is the continued progression of the disease seen in patients who have been started on ATT. This has been postulated to be due to release of antigens from the dying bacilli. These patients require an increased dose of systemic steroids/immunosuppressive therapy to prevent damage to ocular tissues due to excessive release of inflammatory mediators. It is important for clinicians to be aware of this phenomenon and continue patients on ATT despite initial worsening as it can help in decreasing recurrences in long-term follow-up [41, 48]. Intravitreal injections of methotrexate or dexamethasone implant, too, have been reported to manage paradoxical worsening (Fig. 1.6) [107–109]; however, the expert committee could not reach any consensus on local therapy, and thus these are left to discretion of treating physicians [103].

Intravitreal anti-vascular endothelial growth factor (anti-VEGF) injections may be used to treat complications of IOTB such as inflammatory choroidal neovascularization or macular edema [42, 60].

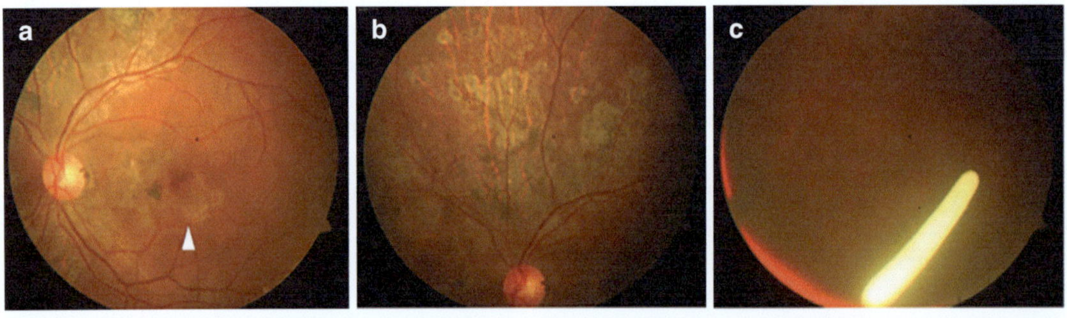

Fig. 1.6 The figure shows a patient with tubercular serpiginous-like choroiditis treated with intravitreal dexamethasone implant (along with anti-tubercular therapy). The fundus photographs with macula in the center (**a**) show active lesions involving the posterior pole (white arrowhead). The superior retina shows healed inactive lesions (**b**). The intravitreal dexamethasone implant injection is seen in the inferior vitreous cavity (**c**)

Conclusion

It is important to have a high index of suspicion based on the history and phenotype. The patients with characteristic phenotype and corroborative evidence of TB may be initiated ATT. That helps in reducing the recurrence.

Compliance with Ethical Requirements The authors declare that they have no conflicts of interest.

References

1. Gupta V, Gupta A, Rao NA. Intraocular tuberculosis—an update. Surv Ophthalmol. 2007;52:561–87. https://doi.org/10.1016/j.survophthal.2007.08.015.
2. World Health Organization. WHO | Global tuberculosis report 2019. WHO n.d.. http://www.who.int/tb/publications/global_report/en/ (accessed October 9, 2020).
3. Helm CJ, Holland GN. Ocular tuberculosis. Surv Ophthalmol. 1993;38:229–56. https://doi.org/10.1016/0039-6257(93)90076-J.
4. Donahue HC. Ophthalmologic experience in a tuberculosis sanatorium. Am J Ophthalmol. 1967; https://doi.org/10.1016/0002-9394(67)92860-7.
5. Bouza E, Merino P, Muñoz P, Sanchez-Carrillo C, Yáñez J, Cortés C. Ocular tuberculosis a prospective study in a general hospital. Medicine (Baltimore). 1997; https://doi.org/10.1097/00005792-199701000-00005.
6. Beare NAV, Kublin JG, Lewis DK, Schijffelen MJ, Peters RPH, Joaki G, et al. Ocular disease in patients with tuberculosis and HIV presenting with fever in Africa. Br J Ophthalmol. 2002; https://doi.org/10.1136/bjo.86.10.1076.
7. Dalvin LA, Smith WM. Intraocular manifestations of mycobacterium tuberculosis: a review of the literature. J Clin Tuberc Mycobact Dis. 2017;7:13–21. https://doi.org/10.1016/j.jctube.2017.01.003.
8. Testi I, Agrawal R, Mehta S, Basu S, Nguyen Q, Pavesio C, et al. Ocular tuberculosis: where are we today? Indian J Ophthalmol. 2020;68:1808–17. https://doi.org/10.4103/ijo.IJO_1451_20.
9. Gupta V, Shoughy SS, Mahajan S, Khairallah M, Rosenbaum JT, Curi A, et al. Clinics of ocular tuberculosis. Ocul Immunol Inflamm. 2015;23:14–24. https://doi.org/10.3109/09273948.2014.986582.
10. Agrawal R, Gunasekeran DV, Grant R, Agarwal A, Kon OM, Nguyen QD, et al. Clinical features and outcomes of patients with tubercular uveitis treated with antitubercular therapy in the collaborative ocular tuberculosis study (COTS)-1. JAMA Ophthalmol. 2017;135:1318–27. https://doi.org/10.1001/jamaophthalmol.2017.4485.
11. Agrawal R, Gunasekeran DV, Raje D, Agarwal A, Nguyen QD, Kon OM, et al. Global variations and challenges with tubercular uveitis in the collaborative ocular tuberculosis study. Invest Ophthalmol Vis Sci. 2018;59:4162–71. https://doi.org/10.1167/iovs.18-24102.
12. Agarwal A, Aggarwal K, Gupta V. Infectious uveitis: an Asian perspective. Eye Lond Engl. 2019;33:50–65. https://doi.org/10.1038/s41433-018-0224-y.
13. Basu S, Wakefield D, Biswas J, Rao NA. Pathogenesis and pathology of intraocular tuberculosis. Ocul Immunol Inflamm. 2015;23:353–7. https://doi.org/10.3109/09273948.2015.1056536.
14. Hutchinson PE, Kee AR, Agrawal R, Yawata N, Tumulak MJ, Connolly JE, et al. Singapore ocular tuberculosis immunity study (SPOTIS): role of T-lymphocyte profiling in patients with presumed ocular tuberculosis. Ocul Immunol Inflamm. 2020:1–7. https://doi.org/10.1080/09273948.2020.1767791.
15. Basu S, Fowler BJ, Kerur N, Arnvig KB, Rao NA. NLRP3 inflammasome activation by mycobacterial ESAT-6 and dsRNA in intraocular tuberculosis. Microb Pathog. 2018;114:219–24. https://doi.org/10.1016/j.micpath.2017.11.044.
16. Albert DM, Raven ML. Ocular tuberculosis historical considerations. 2017;4:1–36. https://doi.org/10.1128/microbiolspec.TNMI7-0001-2016.
17. Abhishek S, Ryndak MB, Choudhary A, Sharma S, Gupta A, Gupta V, et al. Transcriptional signatures of Mycobacterium tuberculosis in mouse model of intraocular tuberculosis. Pathog Dis. 2019:77. https://doi.org/10.1093/femspd/ftz045.
18. Alcolea A, Suarez MJ, Lizasoain M, Tejada P, Chaves F, Palenque E. Conjunctivitis with regional lymphadenopathy in a trainee microbiologist. J Clin Microbiol. 2009; https://doi.org/10.1128/JCM.02253-08.
19. Rohatgi J, Dhaliwal U. Phlyctenular eye disease: a reappraisal. Jpn J Ophthalmol. 2000; https://doi.org/10.1016/S0021-5155(99)00185-9.
20. Bhandari A, Bhandari H, Shukla R, Giri P. Phlyctenular conjunctivitis: a rare association with spinal intramedullary tuberculoma. BMJ Case Rep. 2014; https://doi.org/10.1136/bcr-2013-202010.
21. Ang M, Chee SP. Controversies in ocular tuberculosis. Br J Ophthalmol. 2017; https://doi.org/10.1136/bjophthalmol-2016-309531.
22. Agrawal R, Agarwal A, Jabs DA, Kee A, Testi I, Mahajan S, et al. Standardization of nomenclature for ocular tuberculosis—results of collaborative ocular tuberculosis study (COTS) workshop. Ocul Immunol Inflamm. 2019:1–11. https://doi.org/10.1080/09273948.2019.1653933.
23. Figueira L, Fonseca S, Ladeira I, Duarte R. Ocular tuberculosis: position paper on diagnosis and treatment management. Rev Port Pneumol Engl Ed. 2017;23:31–8. https://doi.org/10.1016/j.rppnen.2016.10.004.

24. Biswas J, Badrinath SS. Ocular morbidity in patients with active systemic tuberculosis. Int Ophthalmol. 1995; https://doi.org/10.1007/BF00130924.
25. Lara LPR, Ocampo V. Prevalence of presumed ocular tuberculosis among pulmonary tuberculosis patients in a tertiary hospital in the Philippines. J Ophthalmic Inflamm Infect. 2013; https://doi.org/10.1186/1869-5760-3-1.
26. Biswas J, Narain S, Das D, Ganesh SK. Pattern of uveitis in a referral uveitis clinic in India. Int Ophthalmol. 1996; https://doi.org/10.1007/bf00175264.
27. Singh R, Gupta V, Gupta A. Pattern of uveitis in a referral eye clinic in North India. Indian J Ophthalmol. 2004;
28. Babu RB, Sudharshan S, Kumarasamy N, Therese L, Biswas J. Ocular tuberculosis in acquired immunodeficiency syndrome. Am J Ophthalmol. 2006; https://doi.org/10.1016/j.ajo.2006.03.062.
29. Gupta A, Sharma A, Bansal R, Sharma K. Classification of intraocular tuberculosis. Ocul Immunol Inflamm. 2015;23:7–13. https://doi.org/10.3109/09273948.2014.967358.
30. Gupta A, Bansal R, Gupta V, Sharma A, Bambery P. Ocular signs predictive of tubercular uveitis. Am J Ophthalmol. 2010; https://doi.org/10.1016/j.ajo.2009.11.020.
31. Sanghvi C, Bell C, Woodhead M, Hardy C, Jones N. Presumed tuberculous uveitis: diagnosis, management, and outcome. Eye. 2011; https://doi.org/10.1038/eye.2010.235.
32. Cordero-Coma M, Calleja S, Torres HE, del Barrio I, Franco M, Yilmaz T, et al. The value of an immune response to Mycobacterium tuberculosis in patients with chronic posterior uveitides revisited: utility of the new IGRAs. Eye. 2010;24:36–43. https://doi.org/10.1038/eye.2009.51.
33. Agrawal R, Betzler B, Testi I, Mahajan S, Agarwal A, Gunasekeran DV, et al. The collaborative ocular tuberculosis study (COTS)-1: a multinational review of 165 patients with tubercular anterior uveitis. Ocul Immunol Inflamm. 2020:1–10. https://doi.org/10.1080/09273948.2020.1761400.
34. Khochtali S, Gargouri S, Abroug N, Ksiaa I, Attia S, Sellami D, et al. The spectrum of presumed tubercular uveitis in Tunisia, North Africa. Int Ophthalmol. 2015;35:663–71. https://doi.org/10.1007/s10792-014-9992-y.
35. Babu K, Bhat SS. Unilateral snow banking in tuberculosis-related intermediate uveitis. J Ophthalmic Inflamm Infect. 2014;4:4. https://doi.org/10.1186/1869-5760-4-4.
36. Parchand S, Tandan M, Gupta V, Gupta A. Intermediate uveitis in Indian population. J Ophthalmic Inflamm Infect. 2011;1:65–70. https://doi.org/10.1007/s12348-011-0020-3.
37. Agarwal A, Afridi R, Agrawal R, Do DV, Gupta V, Nguyen QD. Multimodal imaging in retinal vasculitis. Ocul Immunol Inflamm. 2017;25:424–33. https://doi.org/10.1080/09273948.2017.1319494.
38. Gunasekeran DV, Agrawal R, Agarwal A, Carreño E, Raje D, Aggarwal K, et al. The collaborative ocular tuberculosis study (COTS)-1: a multinational review of 251 patients with tubercular retinal vasculitis. Retina Phila Pa. 2019;39:1623–30. https://doi.org/10.1097/IAE.0000000000002194.
39. Markan A, Aggarwal K, Gupta V, Agarwal A. Bacillary layer detachment in tubercular choroidal granuloma: a new optical coherence tomography finding. Indian J Ophthalmol. 2020;68:1944–6. https://doi.org/10.4103/ijo.IJO_1434_20.
40. Agarwal A, Mahajan S, Khairallah M, Mahendradas P, Gupta A, Gupta V. Multimodal imaging in ocular tuberculosis. Ocul Immunol Inflamm. 2017;25:134–45. https://doi.org/10.1080/09273948.2016.1231332.
41. Arora A, Katoch D, Jain S, Singh SR, Gupta V. Yellow subretinal lesions following initiation of antituberculosis therapy in a tubercular choroidal granuloma: a sign of paradoxical worsening? Ocul Immunol Inflamm. 2020:1–5. https://doi.org/10.1080/09273948.2020.1780272.
42. Jain S, Agarwal A, Gupta V. Resolution of large choroidal tuberculoma following monotherapy with intravitreal ranibizumab. Ocul Immunol Inflamm. 2020;28:494–7. https://doi.org/10.1080/09273948.2019.1582786.
43. Aggarwal K, Agarwal A, Sehgal S, Sharma S, Singh N, Sharma K, et al. An unusual presentation of intraocular tuberculosis in a monocular patient: clinicopathological correlation. J Ophthalmic Inflamm Infect. 2016;6:46. https://doi.org/10.1186/s12348-016-0118-8.
44. Nair N, Sudharshan S, Ram Prakash M, Khetan V, Rao C. Tubercular subretinal abscess in a pediatric intermediate uveitis patient on methotrexate. Indian J Ophthalmol. 2020;68:2043–5. https://doi.org/10.4103/ijo.IJO_362_20.
45. Shetty SB, Bawtag MA, Biswas J. A case of subretinal tubercular abscess presenting as disc edema. Indian J Ophthalmol. 2015;63:164–6. https://doi.org/10.4103/0301-4738.154405.
46. Bansal R, Gupta A, Gupta V, Dogra MR, Sharma A, Bambery P. Tubercular serpiginous-like choroiditis presenting as multifocal serpiginoid choroiditis. Ophthalmology. 2012;119:2334–42. https://doi.org/10.1016/j.ophtha.2012.05.034.
47. Gupta V, Gupta A, Arora S, Bambery P, Dogra MR, Agarwal A. Presumed tubercular serpiginouslike choroiditis: clinical presentations and management. Ophthalmology. 2003;110:1744–9. https://doi.org/10.1016/S0161-6420(03)00619-5.
48. Gupta V, Bansal R, Gupta A. Continuous progression of tubercular serpiginous-like choroiditis after initiating antituberculosis treatment. Am J Ophthalmol. 2011;152:857–63.e2. https://doi.org/10.1016/j.ajo.2011.05.004.
49. Agarwal A, Aggarwal K, Mandadi SKR, Kumar A, Grewal D, Invernizzi A, et al. Longitudinal follow-up of tubercular serpiginous-like choroiditis

using optical coherence tomography angiography. Retina Phila Pa. 2020; https://doi.org/10.1097/IAE.0000000000002915.
50. Chen L. Tubercular retinal vasculitis. JAMA Ophthalmol. 2019;137:e184499. https://doi.org/10.1001/jamaophthalmol.2018.4499.
51. Agrawal R, Gunasekeran DV, Gonzalez-Lopez JJ, Cardoso J, Gupta B, Addison PKF, et al. Peripheral retinal vasculitis: analysis of 110 consecutive cases and a contemporary reappraisal of tubercular etiology. Retina Phila Pa. 2017;37:112–7. https://doi.org/10.1097/IAE.0000000000001239.
52. Aggarwal K, Mulkutkar S, Mahajan S, Singh R, Sharma A, Bansal R, et al. Role of ultra-wide field imaging in the management of tubercular posterior uveitis. Ocul Immunol Inflamm. 2016;24:631–6. https://doi.org/10.3109/09273948.2015.1099681.
53. Singh R, Toor P, Parchand S, Sharma K, Gupta V, Gupta A. Quantitative polymerase chain reaction for mycobacterium tuberculosis in so-called Eales' disease. Ocul Immunol Inflamm. 2012;20:153–7. https://doi.org/10.3109/09273948.2012.658134.
54. Kharel Sitaula R, Iyer V, Noronha V, Dutta Majumder P, Biswas J. Role of high-resolution computerized tomography chest in identifying tubercular etiology in patients diagnosed as Eales' disease. J Ophthalmic Inflamm Infect. 2017;7:4. https://doi.org/10.1186/s12348-016-0120-1.
55. Majumder PD, Sitaula RK, Biswas J. Pediatric Eales disease: an Indian tertiary eye center experience. J Pediatr Ophthalmol Strabismus. 2018;55:270–4. https://doi.org/10.3928/01913913-20180213-01.
56. Seth PK, Sharma S, Senthil S. Bleb-related tuberculous endophthalmitis following combined phacoemulsification and trabeculectomy with mitomycin C. BMJ Case Rep. 2020:13. https://doi.org/10.1136/bcr-2019-234175.
57. Raina UK, Tuli D, Arora R, Mehta DK, Taneja M. Tubercular endophthalmitis simulating retinoblastoma. Am J Ophthalmol. 2000;130:843–5. https://doi.org/10.1016/s0002-9394(00)00646-2.
58. Sahoo L, Mallick AK, Mohanty G, Swain KP, Nayak S, Sahu AK. Concurrent intramedullary spinal cord and multiple intracranial tuberculomas with tuberculous optic neuritis: a rare case report. Indian J Tuberc. 2017;64:337–40. https://doi.org/10.1016/j.ijtb.2016.10.007.
59. Das JC, Singh K, Sharma P, Singla R. Tuberculous osteomyelitis and optic neuritis. Ophthalmic Surg Lasers Imaging. 2003;34:409–12.
60. Invernizzi A, Franzetti F, Viola F, Meroni L, Staurenghi G. Optic nerve head tubercular granuloma successfully treated with anti-VEGF intravitreal injections in addition to systemic therapy. Eur J Ophthalmol. 2015;25:270–2. https://doi.org/10.5301/ejo.5000528.
61. Agarwal A. Commentary: presumed tubercular posterior scleritis—what is our understanding so far? Indian J Ophthalmol. 2019;67:1365–6. https://doi.org/10.4103/ijo.IJO_732_19.
62. Pappuru RR, Dave VP. An unusual case of ocular tuberculosis presenting as subretinal abscess with posterior scleritis. Int Ophthalmol. 2017;37:285–9. https://doi.org/10.1007/s10792-016-0254-z.
63. Murthy SI, Sabhapandit S, Balamurugan S, Subramaniam P, Sainz-de-la-Maza M, Agarwal M, et al. Scleritis: differentiating infectious from non-infectious entities. Indian J Ophthalmol. 2020;68:1818–28. https://doi.org/10.4103/ijo.IJO_2032_20.
64. Singal A, Aggarwal P, Pandhi D, Rohatgi J. Cutaneous tuberculosis and phlyctenular keratoconjunctivitis: a forgotten association. Indian J Dermatol Venereol Leprol. 2006;72:290–2. https://doi.org/10.4103/0378-6323.26726.
65. Lou SM, Larkin KL, Winthrop K, Rosenbaum JT, Accorinti M, Androudi S, et al. Lack of consensus in the diagnosis and treatment for ocular tuberculosis among uveitis specialists. Ocul Immunol Inflamm. 2015;23:25–31. https://doi.org/10.3109/09273948.2014.926936.
66. Lou SM, Montgomery PA, Larkin KL, Winthrop K, Zierhut M, Rosenbaum JT, et al. Diagnosis and treatment for ocular tuberculosis among uveitis specialists: the international perspective. Ocul Immunol Inflamm. 2015;23:32–9. https://doi.org/10.3109/09273948.2014.994784.
67. Mechal Y, Benaissa E, El mrimar N, Benlahlou Y, Bssaibis F, Zegmout A, et al. Evaluation of GeneXpert MTB/RIF system performances in the diagnosis of extrapulmonary tuberculosis. BMC Infect Dis. 2019;19:1069. https://doi.org/10.1186/s12879-019-4687-7.
68. Biswas J, Madhavan HN, Gopal L, Badrinath SS. Intraocular tuberculosis: clinicopathologic study of five cases. Retina. 1995;15:461–8. https://doi.org/10.1097/00006982-199515060-00001.
69. Wroblewski KJ, Hidayat AA, Neafie RC, Rao NA, Zapor M. Ocular tuberculosis: a clinicopathologic and molecular study. Ophthalmology. 2011;118:772–7. https://doi.org/10.1016/j.ophtha.2010.08.011.
70. Biswas J, Kazi MS, Agarwal VA, Alam MS, Therese KL. Polymerase chain reaction for mycobacterium tuberculosis DNA detection from ocular fluids in patients with various types of choroiditis in a referral eye center in India. Indian J Ophthalmol. 2016;64:904–7. https://doi.org/10.4103/0301-4738.198857.
71. Kotake S, Kimura K, Yoshikawa K, Sasamoto Y, Matsuda A, Nishikawa T, et al. Polymerase chain reaction for the detection of Mycobacterium tuberculosis in ocular tuberculosis. Am J Ophthalmol. 1994;117:805–6. https://doi.org/10.1016/s0002-9394(14)70328-9.
72. Agarwal A, Agrawal R, Gunasekaran DV, Raje D, Gupta B, Aggarwal K, et al. The collaborative ocular tuberculosis study (COTS)-1 report 3: polymerase chain reaction in the diagnosis and management of tubercular uveitis: global trends. Ocul Immunol Inflamm. 2019;27:465–73. https://doi.org/10.1080/09273948.2017.1406529.

73. Agarwal A, Marchese A, Rabiolo A, Agrawal R, Bansal R, Gupta V. Clinical and imaging factors associated with the outcomes of tubercular serpiginous-like choroiditis. Am J Ophthalmol. 2020; https://doi.org/10.1016/j.ajo.2020.07.024.
74. Bansal R, Kulkarni P, Gupta A, Gupta V, Dogra MR. High-resolution spectral domain optical coherence tomography and fundus autofluorescence correlation in tubercular serpiginouslike choroiditis. J Ophthalmic Inflamm Infect. 2011;1:157–63. https://doi.org/10.1007/s12348-011-0037-7.
75. Gupta A, Bansal R, Gupta V, Sharma A. Fundus autofluorescence in serpiginouslike choroiditis. Retina Phila Pa. 2012;32:814–25. https://doi.org/10.1097/IAE.0b013e3182278c41.
76. Marchese A, Agarwal A, Moretti AG, Handa S, Modorati G, Querques G, et al. Advances in imaging of uveitis. Ther Adv Ophthalmol. 2020;12:2515841420917781. https://doi.org/10.1177/2515841420917781.
77. Cimino L, Auer C, Herbort CP. Sensitivity of indocyanine green angiography for the follow-up of active inflammatory choriocapillaropathies. Ocul Immunol Inflamm. 2000;8:275–83. https://doi.org/10.1076/ocii.8.4.275.6462.
78. Mandadi SKR, Agarwal A, Aggarwal K, Moharana B, Singh R, Sharma A, et al. Novel findings on optical coherence tomography angiography in patients with tubercular serpiginous-like choroiditis. Retina Phila Pa. 2017;37:1647–59. https://doi.org/10.1097/IAE.0000000000001412.
79. Agarwal A, Agrawal R, Khandelwal N, Invernizzi A, Aggarwal K, Sharma A, et al. Choroidal structural changes in tubercular multifocal Serpiginoid choroiditis. Ocul Immunol Inflamm. 2018;26:838–44. https://doi.org/10.1080/09273948.2017.1370650.
80. Invernizzi A, Mapelli C, Viola F, Cigada M, Cimino L, Ratiglia R, et al. Choroidal granulomas visualized by enhanced depth imaging optical coherence tomography. Retina Phila Pa. 2015;35:525–31. https://doi.org/10.1097/IAE.0000000000000312.
81. Invernizzi A, Agarwal A, Mapelli C, Nguyen QD, Staurenghi G, Viola F. Longitudinal follow-up of choroidal granulomas using enhanced depth imaging optical coherence tomography. Retina Phila Pa. 2017;37:144–53. https://doi.org/10.1097/IAE.0000000000001128.
82. Klufas MA, Phasukkijwatana N, Iafe NA, Prasad PS, Agarwal A, Gupta V, et al. Optical coherence tomography angiography reveals choriocapillaris flow reduction in placoid chorioretinitis. Ophthalmol Retina. 2017;1:77–91. https://doi.org/10.1016/j.oret.2016.08.008.
83. Menzies D, Pai M, Comstock G. Meta-analysis: new tests for the diagnosis of latent tuberculosis infection: areas of uncertainty and recommendations for research. Ann Intern Med. 2007;146:340. https://doi.org/10.7326/0003-4819-146-5-200703060-00006.
84. Ang M, Htoon HM, Chee S-P. Diagnosis of tuberculous uveitis: clinical application of an interferon-gamma release assay. Ophthalmology. 2009;116:1391–6. https://doi.org/10.1016/j.ophtha.2009.02.005.
85. Babu K, Satish V, Satish S, SubbaKrishna D, Abraham M, Murthy K. Utility of QuantiFERON TB gold test in a south Indian patient population of ocular inflammation. Indian J Ophthalmol. 2009;57:427. https://doi.org/10.4103/0301-4738.57147.
86. Pai M, Joshi R, Dogra S, Mendiratta DK, Narang P, Kalantri S, et al. Serial testing of health care workers for tuberculosis using interferon-γ assay. Am J Respir Crit Care Med. 2006;174:349–55. https://doi.org/10.1164/rccm.200604-472OC.
87. Slater ML, Welland G, Pai M, Parsonnet J, Banaei N. Challenges with QuantiFERON-TB gold assay for large-scale, routine screening of U.S. healthcare workers. Am J Respir Crit Care Med. 2013;188:1005–10. https://doi.org/10.1164/rccm.201305-0831OC.
88. Gineys R, Bodaghi B, Carcelain G, Cassoux N, Boutin LTH, Amoura Z, et al. QuantiFERON-TB gold cut-off value: implications for the management of tuberculosis-related ocular inflammation. Am J Ophthalmol. 2011;152:433–40.e1. https://doi.org/10.1016/j.ajo.2011.02.006.
89. La Distia NR, van Velthoven MEJ, ten Dam-van Loon NH, Misotten T, Bakker M, van Hagen MP, et al. Clinical manifestations of patients with intraocular inflammation and positive QuantiFERON–TB gold in-tube test in a country nonendemic for tuberculosis. Am J Ophthalmol. 2014;157:754–61. https://doi.org/10.1016/j.ajo.2013.11.013.
90. Ang M, Hedayatfar A, Wong W, Chee S-P. Duration of anti-tubercular therapy in uveitis associated with latent tuberculosis: a case–control study. Br J Ophthalmol. 2012;96:332–6. https://doi.org/10.1136/bjophthalmol-2011-300209.
91. Shaw JA, Smit DP, Griffith-Richards S, Koegelenberg CFN. Utility of routine chest radiography in ocular tuberculosis and sarcoidosis. Int J Tuberc Lung Dis. 2018; https://doi.org/10.5588/ijtld.18.0013.
92. Petrushkin H, Sethi C, Potter J, Martin L, Russell G, White V, et al. Developing a pathway for the diagnosis and management of ocular tuberculosis. The pan-LOndon ocular tuberculosis pathway—LOOP. Eye. 2020;34:805–8. https://doi.org/10.1038/s41433-019-0543-7.
93. Krassas N, Wells J, Bell C, Woodhead M, Jones N. Presumed tuberculosis-associated uveitis: rising incidence and widening criteria for diagnosis in a non-endemic area. Eye. 2018;32:87–92. https://doi.org/10.1038/eye.2017.152.
94. Manousaridis K, Ong E, Stenton C, Gupta R, Browning AC, Pandit R. Clinical presentation, treatment, and outcomes in presumed intraocular tuberculosis: experience from Newcastle upon Tyne, UK. Eye. 2013;27:480–6. https://doi.org/10.1038/eye.2013.11.
95. Ng KK, Nisbet M, Damato EM, Sims JL. Presumed tuberculous uveitis in non-endemic country for

tuberculosis: case series from a New Zealand tertiary uveitis clinic: tuberculous uveitis in Auckland. Clin Exp Ophthalmol. 2017;45:357–65. https://doi.org/10.1111/ceo.12881.
96. Teixeira-Lopes F, Alfarroba S, Dinis A, Gomes MC, Tavares A. Ocular tuberculosis—a closer look to an increasing reality. Pulmonology. 2018;24:289–93. https://doi.org/10.1016/j.pulmoe.2018.02.006.
97. Bansal R, Gupta A, Gupta V, Dogra MR, Bambery P, Arora SK. Role of anti-tubercular therapy in uveitis with latent/manifest tuberculosis. Am J Ophthalmol. 2008;146:772–9. https://doi.org/10.1016/j.ajo.2008.06.011.
98. Agarwal A, Agrawal R, Raje D, Testi I, Mahajan S, Gunasekeran DV, et al. Twenty-four month outcomes in the collaborative ocular tuberculosis study (COTS)-1: defining the "cure" in ocular tuberculosis. Ocul Immunol Inflamm. 2020:1–9. https://doi.org/10.1080/09273948.2020.1761401.
99. Cunningham ET, Gupta A, Zierhut M. The creeping Choroiditides—serpiginous and multifocal serpiginoid choroiditis. Ocul Immunol Inflamm. 2014;22:345–8. https://doi.org/10.3109/09273948.2014.962924.
100. Nazari Khanamiri H, Rao NA. Serpiginous choroiditis and infectious multifocal serpiginoid choroiditis. Surv Ophthalmol. 2013;58:203–32. https://doi.org/10.1016/j.survophthal.2012.08.008.
101. Grosse V, Bange F, Tischendorf J, Schmidt R, Manns M. A mass in the eye. Lancet. 2002;360:922. https://doi.org/10.1016/S0140-6736(02)11029-4.
102. Lee C, Agrawal R, Pavesio C. Ocular tuberculosis—a clinical conundrum. Ocul Immunol Inflamm. 2015:1–6. https://doi.org/10.3109/09273948.2014.985387.
103. Agrawal R, Testi I, Mahajan S, Yuen YS, Agarwal A, Kon OM, et al. Collaborative ocular tuberculosis study consensus guidelines on the management of tubercular uveitis-report 1: guidelines for initiating antitubercular therapy in tubercular choroiditis. Ophthalmology. 2020; https://doi.org/10.1016/j.ophtha.2020.01.008.
104. Agrawal R, Testi I, Bodaghi B, Barisani-Asenbauer T, McCluskey P, Agarwal A, et al. Collaborative ocular tuberculosis study consensus guidelines on the management of tubercular uveitis-report 2: guidelines for initiating antitubercular therapy in anterior uveitis, intermediate uveitis, panuveitis, and retinal vasculitis. Ophthalmology. 2020; https://doi.org/10.1016/j.ophtha.2020.06.052.
105. Shakarchi F. Ocular tuberculosis: current perspectives. Clin Ophthalmol. 2015:2223. https://doi.org/10.2147/OPTH.S65254.
106. Agrawal R, Gupta B, Gonzalez-Lopez JJ, Rahman F, Phatak S, Triantafyllopoulou I, et al. The role of anti-tubercular therapy in patients with presumed ocular tuberculosis. Ocul Immunol Inflamm. 2015;23:40–6. https://doi.org/10.3109/09273948.2014.986584.
107. Tsui E, Fern CM, Goldberg NR. Treatment of refractory tubercular serpiginous-like choroiditis with intravitreal methotrexate. Retin Cases Brief Rep. 2018; https://doi.org/10.1097/ICB.0000000000000767.
108. Julian K, Langner-Wegscheider B-J, Haas A, De Smet MD. Intravitreal methotrexate in the management of presumed tuberculous serpiginous-like choroiditis. Retina Phila Pa. 2013;33:1943–8. https://doi.org/10.1097/IAE.0b013e318285cdbe.
109. Agarwal A, Handa S, Aggarwal K, Sharma M, Singh R, Sharma A, et al. The role of dexamethasone implant in the management of tubercular uveitis. Ocul Immunol Inflamm. 2018;26:884–92. https://doi.org/10.1080/09273948.2017.1400074.

Nontuberculous Mycobacterial Infections

2

Andrew Zheng, Cyndee Miranda, and Arthi Venkat

Introduction

This chapter will provide a brief introduction to nontuberculous mycobacteria, including organisms involved, types of infections with a particular focus on ocular infections, and risk factors for infection. It will also cover diagnosis and management, particularly the antibiotics used for treatment, as well as side effects and toxicities associated with treatment.

Classification of Non-tuberculous Mycobacteria

The genus *Mycobacterium* includes *M. tuberculosis* complex, *M. leprae*, *M. ulcerans*, and nontuberculous mycobacteria (NTM) [1]. Nontuberculous mycobacteria are a diverse group of organisms, with more than 190 species now identified [1]. Previously, Ernest Runyon classified nontuberculous mycobacteria into four groups based on rate of growth and pigment production [2]. Groups I, II, and III were slowly growing mycobacteria, which usually take 7 days or more to grow in the lab. Group IV were rapidly growing mycobacteria (RGM), which usually grow in less than 7 days. Organisms in Group I (photochromogens) include *M. kansasii*, *M. simiae*, and *M. marinum*. Group II (scotochromogens) include *M. scrofulaceum*, *M. szulgai*, and *M. gordonae*. Group III (nonchromogens) include *M. avium* complex, *M. ulcerans*, *M. xenopi*, *M. malmoense*, *M. terrae* complex, *M. haemophilum*, and *M. genavense*. Group IV (RGM) include *M. abscessus* complex, *M. chelonae*, and *M. fortuitum* complex. NTM are found in the environment—in soil and water, including water distribution systems such as household plumbing [3]. NTM can form biofilms and are more likely present in households with water temperature ≤125 °C [3]. NTM have a waxy cell envelope, with lipids comprising up to 60% of the envelope, making them hydrophobic [4, 5]. This enables NTM to resist disinfectants (including chlorine) and antibiotics and allows for surface adherence to solid substrates [2, 5, 6].

A. Zheng
Department of Ophthalmology, Emory University, Atlanta, USA

C. Miranda (✉)
Department of Infectious Diseases, Cleveland Clinic, Cleveland, OH, USA
e-mail: MIRANDC@ccf.org

A. Venkat (✉)
Department of Ophthalmology - Medical Retina and Uveitis, University of Virginia, Charlottesville, USA
e-mail: arthivenkat@virginia.edu

© Springer Nature Switzerland AG 2023
C. Y. Lowder et al. (eds.), *Emerging Ocular Infections*, Essentials in Ophthalmology,
https://doi.org/10.1007/978-3-031-24559-6_2

Ocular Disease Risk Factors and Pathogenesis

NTM are found in soil and water, and infections generally occur through environmental exposures rather than person-to-person or zoonotic transmission. In the eye, inadvertent inoculation via trauma, contact lens use, and refractive or surgical procedures represent major risk factors, and ophthalmic manifestations can differ based on the mode of inoculation or type of surgery.

The most commonly reported cases of NTM infections involve either traumatic or post-procedure endophthalmitis such as that which occurs after cataract surgery, glaucoma tube implant, or intravitreal injection, as well as keratitis after corneal interventions such as laser in situ keratomileusis (LASIK) or keratoplasty [7, 8]. This risk is due in part directly to instrumentation in and around the eye. For example, in a small series of hyperopic patients with post-refractive NTM keratitis, exposure was attributed to a soft contact lens mask used only in hyperopic, but not myopic, LASIK procedures [9].

The risk of ophthalmic surgical procedures for NTM infection is further compounded because these surgeries often involve biomaterials and implants such as intraocular lenses, glaucoma tube shunts, and scleral buckles that serve as a scaffold for biofilm formation. Risk factors that have been identified with NTM ocular infections include history of trauma (superficial or deep penetrating ocular trauma), prior surgery, ocular biomaterials, use of contact lens, procedures such as penetrating keratoplasty and refractive procedures including laser in situ keratomileusis, laser-assisted subepithelial keratectomy, local immunosuppression (topical corticosteroids), and systemic immunosuppression [10, 11].

In a retrospective study of 142 NTM-infected eyes done by Girgis et al., a history of prior ocular surgeries and medications was present in 95.1% of infected eyes, including LASIK, retinal detachment repair, enucleation, cataract extraction with intraocular lens implantation, penetrating keratoplasty or radial keratotomy, and lid repair or blepharoplasty [11]. The study also identified the presence of an implant as a major risk factor for infection that was present in 63% of cases [11]. Implants included prosthetic and orbital floor implants, scleral buckles, dacryocystorhinostomy stents, intraocular lenses, punctal plugs, contact lenses, and glaucoma drainage implants. Systemic disease was identified in 2.8% and 1.4% had HIV infection. In 76.6% of eyes, use of topical or systemic steroids was identified [11]. Moreover, the glycocalyx surrounding the biofilm lends further adherence and mechanical resistance to host immune responses, thereby rendering the pathogen very difficult to treat once it has established itself within the eye [12, 13]. In 19 patients identified by Shah et al., endophthalmitis caused by NTM occurred in the setting of post-cataract surgery, post-glaucoma implant, post-intravitreal injection, endogenous endophthalmitis, post-pars plana vitrectomy, and post-scleral buckle exposure [7]. Postoperative NTM endophthalmitis was described by Hsu et al. occurring in nine cases after cataract surgery [14]. *M. chelonae*/*M. abscessus* was cultured from intraocular fluid (either aqueous humor or vitreous fluid, or both) in all of the nine cases [14].

NTM intraocular infections have been observed to be increasing in prevalence over recent decades and are likely to become more clinically relevant and significant as both surgical volume and diversity of intraocular implants continue to increase [11].

Endogenous seeding of the eye from a systemic infection can also be seen in a variety of NTM species. However, systemic NTM infection is relatively uncommon in healthy individuals, and infected patients generally have either suppressed immunity, due to either medications or illness, or procedures (especially open-heart surgery) that expose them to large inoculums of the pathogen. One of the earliest reports of NTM endophthalmitis was in a diabetic, post-transplant patient on immunomodulatory therapy (IMT) who developed *M. chelonae* infection from a foot ulcer which spread endogenously to the eye shortly thereafter [15]. More recently, an international outbreak of *M. chimaera* infection after open-heart surgeries has been associated with water droplet exposure from contaminated operating room heating and cooling units [16]; many of these patients then go on to develop a bilateral multifocal choroiditis [17].

Clinical Features

NTM can infect the eyes as a primary infection or may affect the eye by dissemination from another focus of infection.

Ocular Infections

NTM ocular infections can involve all ocular tissues [10]. Although rare, the incidence of NTM ophthalmic infections has increased, with most cases related to surgical complications or trauma [18]. NTM infections include periocular and adnexal infections (eyelids and periocular skin, dacryocystitis, canaliculitis, orbital infections), external ocular infections (conjunctivitis, scleritis, keratitis), and intraocular infections (endophthalmitis) [10]. Rapidly growing mycobacteria are most commonly implicated. Girgis et al. looked at 139 patients with culture-confirmed nontuberculous mycobacteria from 1980 to July 2007 [11]. *M. abscessus/chelonae* was found in 83% of isolates, followed by *M. fortuitum* and *M. avium* complex. Most common infections included keratitis, scleral buckle infections, and socket/implant infections [11]. Chu et al. identified 39 patients with culture-proven NTM ocular infections in Taiwan [19]. Twenty-four isolates were available for molecular identification, with 19 isolates identified as *M. abscessus* group (10 reclassified as *M. abscessus* and the remaining 9 were *M. massiliense*). Infections identified were scleritis, scleral buckle infection, and canaliculitis [19]. A retrospective study of endophthalmitis by Shah et al. identified 19 patients with endophthalmitis, with *M. chelonae* identified in 14 patients and *M. fortuitum* in 3 patients [7].

Ocular Adnexal and Orbital Infection

NTM infections of ocular adnexal structures can present as preseptal cellulitis of the periocular skin, canaliculitis, or dacryocystitis, with characteristic pain, redness, swelling, induration, and/or mucopurulent discharge [10]. In some cases, external dacryocystorhinostomy (DCR) scars of the skin overlying the lacrimal sac can be found, suggesting a possible infectious source either from chronic nasolacrimal duct obstruction (NLDO) or prior surgery. In other cases, there may be underlying immune compromise—such as from diabetes, medications, malignancy, or human immunodeficiency virus (HIV).

Orbital infection with NTM is rare but has been reported mostly in the setting of trauma and surgery, including two cases which occurred on the orbital implant after enucleation [20]. In some cases the infection may present as an intraconal or retroseptal mass or abscess visible on orbital imaging studies, and the disease course can be variable and dependent on the nature of the underlying injury. In their review of eight cases published in the literature, Moorthy et al. report that patients generally experience periorbital edema without significant proptosis lasting anywhere from 2 weeks to 11 months, with visual outcomes that range from normal to no light perception (NLP) [10]. As with any orbital process, ocular motility defects can be seen but are generally subtle in the context of NTM infections. Fast-growing Runyon group IV organisms including *M. abscessus*, *M. chelonae*, and *M. fortuitum* are the causative pathogen in almost all ocular adnexal and orbital infections.

Conjunctivitis and Scleritis

As with orbital infections, NTM-associated conjunctivitis and scleritis are rare but have been reported to occur after intraocular surgery and scleral buckling, with highly variable disease course and outcomes. Oz et al. reported a case of NTM infection in a patient with a scleral buckle (SB) implanted 18 years prior, who presented with mild anterior uveitis and conjunctival hyperemia and thinning that progressed over 5 months to erosion and SB exposure [21]. Subsequent SB explantation and culture demonstrated *M. chelo-*

nae, and the patient did well after a course of topical antibiotics and steroids. Others cases have been more severe, with reports of scleral abscesses, thinning, and, in several cases, perforation leading to removal of the eye [22–24]. Often patients will have subconjunctival nodules representing active sites of bacterial inflammation, which may recur or progress towards deeper and more extensive involvement despite aggressive antibiotic therapy, debridement, and surgery. In at least one case, infection progressed to involve the cornea despite good antimicrobial control of the primary conjunctival and scleral sites of infection [23]. Almost all reported cases of NTM conjunctivitis and scleritis are due to the same group IV fast-growing mycobacteria seen in orbital and ocular adnexal infections, *M. chelonae*, *M. abscessus*, and *M. fortuitum.*

Keratitis

Corneal infection, often occurring after trauma, refractive surgery, or keratoplasty, represents a common manifestation of ocular NTM disease. As with most other manifestations of ocular-involving NTM infection, the causative pathogens are predominantly Runyon group IV organisms (*M. chelonae*, *M. abscessus*, and *M. fortuitum*), although rare cases of infection by group II organisms (*M. gordonae*) have also been reported [25]. Onset is usually delayed, with symptoms generally presenting 2–3 weeks after the inciting surgery or trauma, although symptom onset as soon as 3 days and as late as 1 year afterwards has been reported [8, 13]. Patients present with decreased vision, redness, photophobia, and pain that is generally moderate and less severe than that seen in *Acanthamoeba* infections. On examination, anterior uveitis is common, and epithelial defects, stromal infiltrates, crystalline keratopathy, or frank corneal ulceration can also be seen [8, 26]. In later stages of disease, corneal scarring and thinning are common although, in contrast to NTM-associated scleritis, perforation is unusual and enucleation is rarely necessary.

Endophthalmitis

NTM can also cause both endogenous and exogenous endophthalmitis; the group IV organisms *M. chelonae*, *M. abscessus*, and *M. fortuitum* are often implicated, although *M. avium-intracellulare* complex (MAC) has also been reported [7]. Endogenous seeding is relatively less common than exogenous endophthalmitis and is seen almost exclusively in the context of immunosuppression; one of the earliest reports of NTM endophthalmitis, for example, was described in a diabetic post-renal transplant patient on IMT who subsequently became septic from a diabetic foot ulcer and seeded mycobacteria to the left eye [15]. Most reported cases of exogenous endophthalmitis occur after intraocular surgery involving implanted devices—typically cataract extraction with intraocular lens, glaucoma tube insertion, or rarely lamellar corneal transplantation [13, 27–29]. However, a few cases of post-injection and post-pars plana vitrectomy (PPV) infection have been noted as well [7]. Coincidentally, many exogenous endophthalmitis patients also have concomitant immunosuppressed states that may potentiate their susceptibility to infection. Patients present with typical findings of anterior chamber inflammation with or without hypopyon, as well as vitritis, generally 3 to 8 weeks after surgery. A biofilm can be commonly found growing over implanted materials and devices either at the time of diagnosis or during subsequent therapeutic surgeries. Infection and inflammation may extend and go on to involve other ocular structures including the cornea and sclera and may cause hypotony, retinal detachment (RD), or globe perforation [7, 27, 28].

The differential diagnosis of NTM-associated endophthalmitis includes other causes of chronic endophthalmitis such as *Cutibacterium (*formerly *Propionibacterium) acnes*, *Corynebacterium* species, *Nocardia*, or fungal infection. Due to this broad differential and its relative rarity, NTM is often initially overlooked as a cause of postoperative chronic infection. In one series of 19 patients, the mean time from symptom onset to diagnosis was 9 weeks [7]. This delay in diagnosis, coupled with often serious late sequelae of infection, contributes to generally poor visual outcomes in NTM endophthalmitis. Among several series and case reports, a majority of patients have a final BCVA of less than 20/400, and approximately one-fifth of patients progress towards phthisis or enucleation [7, 27, 29].

Chorioretinitis

Systemic opportunistic NTM infections in late-stage AIDS patients are well-known, generally involving group III MAC species, and several reports have documented disseminated infection to the eye [30, 31]. Posterior findings can be prominent in these cases, often presenting as a multifocal granulomatous process in the choroid [32–34].

There had also been rare isolated cases of NTM choroiditis in immunocompetent patients [35], but until recently, this phenotype of NTM ocular infection was seen almost exclusively in severely immunocompromised patients, many of whom died shortly after diagnosis. Thus, detailed descriptions of clinical course and outcomes in these cases had been lacking. In 2017 however, a number of open-heart surgery patients with systemic postoperative infections of *M. chimaera*—a close relative of MAC—were found to have bilateral multifocal choroiditis. In contrast to previously reported cases of MAC or NTM chorioretinitis, all patients within this cardiac surgery cohort were HIV negative, and the majority were not on IMT [17, 36]. Choroidal lesions ranged in size from 50 to 1100 μm in diameter, with variable number and extent throughout the fundus which correlated directly with the severity and extent of systemic infection. Associated ocular findings included anterior and intermediate uveitis and optic nerve head swelling. Although it was a disseminated disease, chorioretinitis was an important clinical finding in the *M. chimaera* infection outbreak. Two cases of choroiditis were reported in the series by Scriven et al. [37], and Boni et al. [36] found nine male patients with choroidal lesions. In the six patients initially identified in Zurich, five patients had ocular findings, including mild anterior and intermediate uveitis, optic disc swelling, and white-yellowish choroidal lesions suggestive of chorioretinitis [17]. All of the patients were diagnosed with endocarditis or aortic graft infection. Two patients had few choroidal lesions, while three patients had more severe and progressive bilateral multifocal choroiditis. The three patients with progressive ocular disease died, with pathology of one of the patients showing prominent patchy lymphohistiocytic and granulomatous choroiditis. These findings indicated that severity of ocular involvement correlated with systemic disease severity [17]. Four additional cases were later identified as having ocular involvement with *M. chimaera*—two with more extensive multifocal choroiditis and two with fewer choroidal lesions [36]. Of these nine patients with ocular findings, two had vision changes at baseline, and the rest were asymptomatic. However, two of the patients who did not have visual symptoms at baseline later developed decreased vision and blurriness [36]. In a report of three cases with fatal, disseminated *M. chimaera* with active granulomatous encephalitis, all three patients had choroidal granulomas [38]. Therefore, ophthalmologic examination should be done in all patients suspected with disseminated *M. chimaera*, even in those without any visual complaints [38, 39].

Extraocular Infections

Most extraocular NTM infections are pulmonary. Pulmonary NTM disease is much more common than ocular NTM disease. In pulmonary disease, the most common NTM pathogens are *M. avium* complex, *M. kansasii*, *M. xenopi*, and *M. abscessus* [1]. NTM lung disease occurs in patients with anatomic lung disease, in patients with immunologic or genetic predisposition/abnormalities, and in patients with no underlying lung or immunologic abnormalities [4]. *Mycobacterium avium* complex pulmonary disease is an interplay between environmental exposure, host susceptibility, and pathogen virulence [40]. In general, there is no human-to-human transmission, except in transmission that was described in cystic fibrosis patients with *M. abscessus* [2]. The incidence of NTM lung disease has been increasing. Winthrop et al. found an increase in the annual incidence of NTM from 3.13 to 4.73 per 100,000 person-years from 2008 to 2015, using administrative claims-based NTM lung disease in a US-managed care claims database [41]. The annual prevalence increased from 6.78 to 11.70 per 100,000 persons [41]. NTM lung disease can present as nodular bronchiectatic disease, fibrocavitary disease, and hypersensitivity pneumonitis [42].

NTM can also cause other extrapulmonary diseases, including lymphadenitis, skin and soft tissue infections, bone infections, central nervous system infections, and disseminated disease. Skin and soft tissue infections are the most common extrapulmonary NTM infections [18]. Rapidly growing mycobacteria such as *M. abscessus*, *M. chelonae*, and *M. fortuitum* usually cause skin lesions at puncture wounds, open injuries due to trauma, or fractures [6]. Lower extremity folliculitis caused by rapidly growing mycobacteria has also been reported with the use of contaminated nail salon whirlpool footbaths [43]. Tattooing has also been associated with infection with *M. chelonae* [18]. Healthcare-associated outbreaks and pseudo-outbreaks have also been described, including those associated with cardiac surgery, liposuction, plastic surgeries, LASIK, injections, and central line-related infections, presumably due to NTM-infected liquid such as tap water [6]. Other healthcare-associated infections include those associated with prosthetic devices, including prosthetic heart valves, lens implants, artificial hips and knees, and metal rods for fractures [43]. Investigators in Brazil reported an epidemic of RGM infection occurring after video-assisted surgery with 1051 possible cases from 2006 to 2007 in Rio de Janeiro [44]. The RGM was identified as *M. massiliense*. The Centers for Disease Control also reported on RGM infections in medical tourists returning from Dominican Republic after cosmetic surgery procedures such as liposuction, abdominoplasty, and breast implantations [45]. Contaminated ultrasound gel, injection of dermal fillers, mesotherapy, and acupuncture have also been associated with outbreaks [18].

Disseminated disease is usually seen in those with underlying immunosuppression, such as organ transplant recipients, patients on tumor necrosis factor inhibitors, patients with AIDS, and those with Mendelian susceptibility to mycobacterial disease [4]. Disseminated *Mycobacterium avium* complex (most commonly due to *M. avium*) occurs in patients with untreated AIDS [6, 40]. Rapidly growing mycobacteria such as *M. abscessus* and *M. chelonae* can also cause disseminated infection in immunosuppressed patients [6].

As described earlier in this chapter, a global outbreak of disseminated *M. chimaera* has been described in patients who have undergone cardiac surgery, related to heater-cooler unit contamination [39]. In 2015, a cluster of six patients with invasive *M. chimaera* infection among those who had undergone open-heart surgery was reported by investigators in Switzerland [46]. *M. chimaera* is one of the species in the *Mycobacterium avium* complex, and more than 100 cases of disseminated infection have been reported worldwide in connection with this outbreak [39]. The outbreak has been due to exposure to contaminated heater-cooler units manufactured by LivaNova PLC used during cardiopulmonary bypass, with *M. chimaera* aerosolized from these devices during surgery [46]. Later investigation revealed that contamination of heater-cooler units most likely occurred during production in Germany [46]. This outbreak has high mortality rates (46%) and as high as 63% in the outbreak reported in Pennsylvania [39]. Some of the laboratory findings include cytopenias, transaminitis, elevated markers of inflammation, and elevated creatinine [39]. Scriven et al. described *M. chimaera* infection following cardiac surgery in the UK, with 30 cases identified [37]. Most common clinical findings included fever, malaise, weight loss, cough, dyspnea, and splenomegaly [37]. Prosthetic valve endocarditis (PVE) was seen in 38% of patients, including three patients who initially had normal echocardiography and later showed evidence of PVE [37]. Aortic graft infection and chronic sternal wound infection were also described [37]. In disseminated infection, most had prosthetic material in place, which included prosthetic valves, vascular grafts, and left ventricular assist devices [39]. Asadi et al. reported two cases of patients who underwent aortic valve surgery and were diagnosed with disseminated *M. chimaera* infection without evidence of prosthetic valve endocarditis [47]. Disseminated infection involved multiple organs in addition to the ophthalmic manifestations described in the previous section, including liver, spleen, bone marrow, spine, skin, and bone [37]. In this particular outbreak, there has been a long latency between clinical presentation and diagnosis, with the longest reported time greater than 6 years from time of surgery to symptoms [39].

Diagnostic Testing

Avoiding delays in diagnosis of NTM infections means having a high index of suspicion and ensuring that appropriate specimens for mycobacterial cultures are sent (acid-fast bacilli smears, cultures, drug susceptibilities) [48]. Diagnosis of NTM in the laboratory is primarily done through mycobacterial culture. Clinical specimens are stained for acid-fast bacilli (usually with fluorochrome), and identifying acid-fast bacilli on smear can mean either NTM or *M. tuberculosis* is present. Nucleic acid amplification tests are useful in rapidly detecting *M. tuberculosis* [40]. Using both solid and liquid media improves the sensitivity of NTM detection [42]. Solid media allow for observation of colony morphology, growth rates, identification of mixed infections, and organism quantitation [6]. Cultures in liquid media are more sensitive and decrease delay in detection of NTM, but are more susceptible to contamination [2]. *M. genavense* and *M. haemophilum* require enrichment of culture media to grow [49]. As not all NTM species are clinically relevant, and NTM species vary in their treatment, accurate identification of NTM species is crucial. Once growth is identified in culture, various methods have been employed for identification. High-performance liquid chromatography (HPLC) has the least ability to discriminate between species and subspecies, and molecular methods have been used more in identification [2]. Line probe assays allow for identification of more commonly encountered NTM species [49]. More precise identification of NTM can be done with gene sequencing. 16S rRNA sequencing can identify to species level, and targets such as *hsp65* and *rpoB* genes can identify to subspecies level [40]. Other methods include real-time PCR, DNA sequencing, and matrix-assisted laser desorption ionization-time of flight (MALDI-TOF) mass spectrometry [2]. Specimens that can be sent for mycobacterial culture include respiratory specimens (sputum or through bronchoscopy), body fluid, abscess fluid, tissue, and blood [6]. It is important to note that swabs are not recommended for mycobacterial culture [6]. It is usually considered clinically significant when NTM is isolated from sterile sites such as blood, tissue, cerebrospinal fluid, pleural fluid, brain, and skin and soft tissue [50, 51].

For ocular infections, aspirates of purulent drainage, conjunctival discharge, exudates or superficial lamellar scleral biopsies and infected scleral buckling explants, corneal scrapings in infectious keratitis, as well as cultures of the anterior chamber and vitreous in patients with NTM endophthalmitis and tissue specimens can be cultured directly [10].

Mycobacterial culture is an important cornerstone of diagnosis and can be utilized for intraocular aqueous or vitreous samples, corneal scrapings, conjunctival and extraocular discharge, and explanted foreign bodies. Middlebrook 7H11 agar or Lowenstein-Jensen medium can be used to selectively grow mycobacteria, but blood agar and MacConkey agar have also been used successfully, especially for the fast-growing group IV organisms that comprise the majority of NTM ocular infections [9, 28]. However, cultures of slow-growing group I, II, and III NTM will take longer than 7 days and in many cases may not grow at all, further delaying diagnosis and appropriate management.

Isolation of NTM from the respiratory tract does not necessarily indicate the presence of pulmonary disease [42], and a single positive sputum culture is not sufficient for formal diagnosis. The American Thoracic Society (ATS) and the Infectious Disease Society of America (IDSA) released a joint statement in 2007 on the diagnosis, treatment, and prevention of nontuberculous mycobacterial infections [6]. Clinical and microbiologic criteria for diagnosis of NTM pulmonary disease were established. Clinical criteria included pulmonary symptoms and nodular or cavitary opacities on chest radiograph or a high-resolution computed tomography scan that shows multifocal bronchiectasis with multiple small nodules and appropriate exclusion of other diagnoses. Microbiologic criteria required positive culture from at least two separate expectorated samples or positive culture from at least one bronchial wash or lavage or transbronchial or other lung biopsy with mycobacterial histopathologic features (granulomatous inflammation or AFB) and positive culture for NTM or biopsy showing mycobacterial histopathologic features (granulomatous inflammation or AFB) and on one or more sputum or bronchial washings that are culture positive for NTM [6]. In July 2020, clinical practice guidelines on the treatment of NTM pulmonary disease were published online, which is now a joint guideline by the ATS, IDSA, the European Respiratory Society (RES), and European Society of Clinical Microbiology and Infectious Diseases (ECSMID) [1]. Decision to treat should be individualized, and meeting diagnostic criteria does not necessarily mean initiating therapy [1].

Diagnostic criteria for pulmonary NTM infections require either two separate positive sputum cultures or positive culture and histopathology results from more invasive bronchial lavage or lung biopsy procedures [6]. Ocular NTM infections are primarily diagnosed via culture or histopathology results based on samples from ocular tissues, but there are no consensus guidelines on the diagnostic gold standard for ocular disease. Moreover, lower clinical suspicion for these rare pathogens and inherent limitations of current diagnostic methods further contribute to delayed diagnoses which are common in cases of NTM ocular infection. As such, most reported cases of NTM-associated eye disease utilize multiple approaches to establish a diagnosis.

An adjunctive diagnostic approach is direct histopathology and microscopy with polymerase chain reaction tests to identify mycobacterial genetic material. The Ziehl-Neelsen acid-fast stain can be used to directly identify mycobacteria within smears of ocular tissue and fluid samples and may be helpful as an alternative method of diagnosis in cases where cultures are non-diagnostic [15, 32]. However, this method may fail to identify as many as two-thirds of all NTM ocular infections since, in the absence of identifiable bacteria, histopathologic features demonstrate mostly nonspecific granulomatous inflammation, necrosis, and foreign-body and Langerhans-type giant cells. Additionally, shared microscopy features with other bacteria may lead to misdiagnosis of NTM species as possibly *Nocardia* (which are weakly acid-fast) or *Corynebacterium* (which are also rod-shaped) [26, 28].

The interferon-gamma release assay (IGRA) is an important screening test that generally distinguishes *M. tuberculosis* (MTB) infection from other NTM infections, and as such it is not widely used for detection of NTM infection specifically. However, there are some data which suggest a degree of cross-reactivity between certain NTM strains and MTB strains, and there is at least one report of *M. kansasii* NTM ocular infection which was incidentally detected on IGRA screening and confirmed via bronchial aspirate [35, 52]. This overlap may be particularly relevant in certain cases, as IGRA and MTB infection are common considerations in a broad range of uveitis evaluations.

Multimodal ophthalmic imaging also plays a role in the assessment and monitoring of disease, although the nonspecific appearance of NTM infections of the eye renders these tools less useful for establishing a definitive diagnosis. Especially in cases of chorioretinitis, however, imaging allows for a relatively noninvasive and objective means of documenting disease progression and trajectory. Boni et al. evaluated nine patients with *M. chimaera* infection and bilateral choroiditis after open-heart surgery and describe several key features on fundus imaging. First, they note that indocyanine green angiography (ICGA) is superior to other modalities in delineating the extent and number of choroidal lesions, which in turn correlates with and can be used as a proxy for the severity of the underlying systemic infection. With treatment, these hypocyanescent lesions were noted to lighten and become more subtle, but did not resolve completely [36]. They additionally report that on fluorescein angiography (FA), lesions block fluorescence in early frames and stain with hyperfluorescence in late frames, consistent with lesions seen in other outer retinal and choroidal diseases such as sarcoidosis, toxoplasmosis, and many other well-known posterior uveitides. Finally, they also note that imaging can differentiate active fundus lesions, which have ill-defined borders, from inactive ones, which show sharp and discrete outlines.

Management

A broad array of antibiotic classes have been proposed and tried in the management of NTM ocular infections, including aminoglycosides, macrolides, fluoroquinolones, vancomycin, third-generation cephalosporins, carbapenems, and anti-tuberculous regimens. Delivery routes depend in part on the location and extent of infection, although most patients receive combination therapy via multiple different approaches.

Ocular Disease Management

Topical therapy represents the most convenient and least invasive treatment option for many patients, and in cases of isolated keratitis, it may be sufficient as monotherapy [28]. Severity of infection and final visual outcomes in keratitis are variable and depend largely on the nature of the underlying trauma or surgery. For example, infections after refractive surgery, which are generally limited to the LASIK flap interface and the more superficial layers of the cornea, are thought to be milder than that of deeper or penetrating wounds. With few exceptions, final best-corrected visual acuity (BCVA) is generally better, in the range of 20/20 to 20/80 [9, 53]. In contrast, other series of trauma- and keratoplasty-related cases report widely variable BCVA outcomes from 20/20 to hand motion (HM), with over 36% of patients in one series having BCVA of 20/100 or worse [8].

Amikacin and macrolides are often preferred as first-line agents for topical therapy in the eye, although they are relatively uncommon in an ophthalmic eyedrop formulation and may be difficult to obtain [8, 9]. In that regard, topical fluoroquinolones such as ciprofloxacin or ofloxacin can be effective and are commercially available and relatively inexpensive, while fortified vancomycin and ceftazidime may be accessible options through experienced compounding pharmacies. For slower-growing organisms such as *M. gordonae* or *M. kansasii*, topical rifampin may also be acceptable [13, 25]. For more extensive infections that progress to or present as endophthalmitis, intravitreal injections should be considered. In many cases, patients present as undifferentiated chronic endophthalmitis and may often receive empiric therapy with intravitreal vancomycin and ceftazidime for broad coverage. For cases in which diagnosis and causative NTM organism are known, more tailored therapy with intravitreal amikacin 250–400 μg has been discussed, although there is a risk of retinal toxicity from intravitreal aminoglycosides [27, 54].

Surgical intervention and explantation of biomaterials and intraocular devices represent an important facet of NTM ocular infection management. Given the propensity of these organisms for forming biofilms, removal of the nidus and scaffolding for NTM infection is often necessary to achieve a successful cure. Multiple reports have described removal of intraocular lenses, infected SB, and lens capsules as critical steps in the management of intraocular infection [7, 21, 54]. Likewise PPV, therapeutic penetrating keratoplasty, and lamellar keratectomy have all been proposed as a means to debulk or resect en bloc the infected tissue [8, 13, 53].

Systemic Therapy

Systemic, often intravenous (IV), therapy is widely used in the treatment of NTM ocular infections, especially for periocular and orbital infections, scleritis, and endophthalmitis. The course of treatment is often more prolonged compared to treatment for MTB, with regard to both ocular and systemic disease. For example, slow-growing group I and II organisms may be susceptible to four-drug anti-tuberculous therapy, but treatment duration is generally 18 months or double the standard regimen for active MTB [17, 35]. Conventionally, amikacin has been considered first-line therapy for systemic treatment of all NTM, although some data show a 60% rate of resistance to amikacin and ciprofloxacin among certain mycobacterial populations [9]. Recent findings suggest that there is also a difference in antibiotic sensitivities between the less virulent *M. fortuitum* and the more virulent *M. chelonae/abscessus* group. Specifically, *M. fortuitum* is thought to be more sensitive to amikacin and ciprofloxacin, whereas *M. chelonae* may be more effectively treated with clarithromycin [10, 11].

Therapy of NTM differs between species, and thus it is important to identify NTM to species and subspecies level. This information also has implications for treatment outcomes. Therapy of rapidly growing mycobacteria will be discussed first. Clinically relevant RGM species include *M. fortuitum*, *M. chelonae*, and *M. abscessus*. Three subspecies are now identified within the *M. abscessus* complex: *M. abscessus* subspecies *abscessus*, *M. abscessus* subspecies *bolletii*, and *M. abscessus* subspecies *massiliense*. *M. abscessus* is generally the most pathogenic. There are no clinical trials to establish therapy for RGM (except for clarithromycin therapy for *M. chelonae*) [43]. RGM are resistant to first-line anti-tuberculosis agents, and therapeutic agents used are based on unique in vitro susceptibility pattern per species [43]. An important consideration in therapy is that in vitro susceptibilities may not always correlate with clinical response, except for macrolides [48]. Biofilms may contribute to this discrepancy in clinical response [48], as was shown by Greendyke et al. on differential susceptibility of *M. abscessus* variants in biofilms and macrophages [55]. The Clinical and Laboratory Standards Institute (CLSI) recommends drug susceptibility testing for NTM by broth microdilution and in general should be done on clinically relevant isolates [51]. Inducible macrolide resistance must also be taken into account with therapy. Macrolides used in therapy include clarithromycin and azithromycin. Resistance to macrolides can develop through mutations in the 23S rDNA (*rrl*) gene and through the *erm* gene [1]. The *erm* methylase genes confer resistance through reduced binding of macrolides to the ribosomes [50]. Isolates that appear susceptible at day 3 of incubation may no longer be susceptible at day 14 of incubation with macrolides [43]. Most *M. fortuitum* and *M. abscessus* subspecies *abscessus* have the *erm* gene, and *M. chelonae* have no functional erm gene and have little or no change in clarithromycin MICs during extended incubation [43]. *M. abscessus* subspecies *massiliense* also have a dysfunctional *erm* gene [26], and Lee et al. found that most clinical strains of *M. massiliense* were susceptible to clarithromycin [56]. To detect inducible macrolide resistance, CLSI has recommended incubation to 14 days for RGM before final reading of clarithromycin MIC (minimum inhibitory concentration) [43].

CLSI has recommended testing the following antibiotics for RGM: amikacin, cefoxitin, ciprofloxacin, clarithromycin, doxycycline (or minocycline), imipenem, linezolid, moxifloxacin, and trimethoprim-sulfamethoxazole [51]. For *M. chelonae/M. immunogenum* complex, tobramycin is also tested [51]. Other drugs that may also be tested with no established MIC breakpoints include clofazimine (a riminophenazine that has been used in the treatment of leprosy) and tigecycline [43, 51]. In general, treatment involves combination antibiotic therapy. For infections involving prosthetic material, removal of all foreign material is important to achieve cure [48]. For patients with NTM lung disease, surgical resection should be considered in selected patients [40]. In patients with extensive NTM disease, presence of abscesses, drug resistance, or difficulties with drug therapy, surgery should also be considered [48].

For *M. fortuitum*, isolates are generally susceptible to oral agents such as fluoroquinolones (ciprofloxacin, moxifloxacin, levofloxacin), doxycycline, minocycline, sulfonamides, and linezolid [43, 48] and to parenteral agents such as amikacin, cefoxitin, imipenem, and tigecycline [43]. As was discussed earlier, *M. fortuitum* possess the *erm* gene, which confers inducible macrolide resistance. At least two agents with in vitro activity are recommended for treatment [6]. *M. chelonae* are sensitive or intermediate to tobramycin, clarithromycin, linezolid, imipenem, amikacin, clofazimine, doxycycline, ciprofloxacin, and tigecycline [6, 43]. Tobramycin is more active in vitro than amikacin for *M. chelonae*, and isolates are resistant to cefoxitin [6]. Combination drug therapy is also recommended particularly for serious infections involving skin and soft tissue, bone, and lungs, with at least two active agents [6, 48].

Antibiotics used for *M. abscessus* complex include intravenous amikacin, inhaled amikacin, tigecycline, cefoxitin, imipenem, clarithromycin, azithromycin, doxycycline, ciprofloxacin, moxifloxacin, linezolid, and clofazimine [43, 48]. For pulmonary disease, treatment involves an initial phase with parenteral therapy followed by a continuation phase [1]. For strains without inducible macrolide resistance, a regimen that includes a macrolide is recommended, with at least three active agents [1]. For macrolide-resistant strains, a regimen with at least four active agents should be used [1]. Monotherapy is not recommended due to concerns for resistance [48]. Based on the latest ATS/ERS/ECSMID/IDSA clinical practice guideline on the treatment of NTM pulmonary disease by Daley et al., parenteral agents preferred for the initial phase include amikacin, imipenem or cefoxitin, tigecycline (at least 1–2 agents), and an oral antibiotic such as azithromycin, clofazimine, or linezolid [1]. The continuation phase agents include two to three drugs which include azithromycin, clofazimine, linezolid, or inhaled amikacin.

Slowly growing mycobacteria that are known to cause clinical disease include *M. avium* complex (MAC), *M. kansasii*, *M. marinum*, *M. simiae*, *M. scrofulaceum*, *M. szulgai*, *M. gordonae*, *M. ulcerans*, *M. xenopi*, *M. malmoense*, *M. terrae* complex, *M. genavense*, and *M. haemophilum* [2]. Treatment discussion of slowly growing mycobacteria will focus on more common pathogens, namely, *M. avium* complex and *M. kansasii. M. avium* complex consists of multiple species including *M. avium*, *M. intracellulare*, and *M. chimaera*, which are the most significant human pathogens [40]. Other organisms included in MAC are *M. arosiense*, *M. boucherdurhonense*, *M. colombiense*, *M. marseillense*, *M. timonense*, *M. vulneris*, and *M. yongonense* [40]. For *M. avium* complex, macrolides (azithromycin and clarithromycin) are considered the foundation of treatment [1]. In vitro MICs for MAC do not correlate clinically except for macrolides and amikacin [51]. Susceptibilities should only be performed for drugs that show correlation in vitro with microbiologic response, and for MAC, susceptibilities for amikacin and macrolides should be done to guide therapy. Clarithromycin MIC of ≤ 8 is considered susceptible, and MIC ≥ 32 is considered resistant [51]. Amikacin MICs of ≥ 64 is considered resistant for intravenous therapy, and MICs of ≥ 128 is considered resistant for inhaled liposomal amikacin [51]. Based on the latest ATS/ERS/ECSMID/IDSA clinical practice guideline on the treatment of NTM pulmonary disease by Daley et al., treatment regimen for MAC pulmonary disease consists of at least three drugs: azithromycin (if susceptible), ethambutol, and rifampin. Intermittent therapy given three times a week is recommended with nodular/bronchiectatic lung disease, but daily therapy is recommended for cavitary disease, and addition of aminoglycoside (amikacin or streptomycin) is recommended [1]. Inhaled liposomal amikacin may also be used in refractory cases [1]. For macrolide-resistant lung disease, the use of parenteral agents (amikacin or streptomycin) and surgical management have the best treatment outcomes [57]. Alternative agents used for MAC include clofazimine and quinolones [58]. Newer drugs used for NTM treatment include bedaquiline, a diarylquinoline antibiotic that has been used for drug-resistant tuberculosis [51] and has also been used in treatment of MAC [57]. Another new agent is tedizolid, which is another oxazolidinone antibiotic like linezolid and has also been shown to be active against NTM [51].

For extrapulmonary MAC infections, the three-drug regimen with a macrolide should also be used with addition of parenteral aminoglycoside for those with extensive disease or treatment failure [40]. Surgical excision for MAC cervical lymphadenitis is considered first-line therapy [40]. Treatment for skin, soft tissue, tendons, joints, and bones involves medical and surgical therapy such as debridement [6]. Disseminated MAC treatment in patients with HIV/AIDS is treated with clarithromycin and ethambutol, with or without rifabutin [6]. Intravenous amikacin may also be used, but use of clofazimine has previously been associated with increased mortality, although there are other studies that did not find a mortality difference [40]. In disseminated *M. chimaera* infections following cardiac surgery discussed earlier, treatment recommendations differ. A multidrug regimen consisting of four to five antibiotics is recommended, using macrolide, rifamycin, ethambutol, and either moxifloxacin or clofazimine, with possible addition of intravenous amikacin [39]. Removal or exchange of foreign material is recommended, with use of intravenous amikacin before and after surgery in addition to the oral antibiotics [39].

For *M. kansasii*, there is good correlation with in vitro susceptibilities and clinical response, and it is the most easily treatable NTM lung pathogen [58]. Rifampin is an important component for successful therapy [6]. The latest guidelines for treatment of pulmonary disease with *M. kansasii* recommend azithromycin, rifampin, and ethambutol with either daily or intermittent therapy (three times a week) for noncavitary disease and daily therapy for cavitary [1]. Isoniazid can also be used with ethambutol and rifampicin using daily therapy instead of three times weekly. For isolates with rifampin resistance, a flouroquinolone such as moxifloxacin may be used [1]. Other agents that can be used with rifampin resistance include amikacin, linezolid, trimethoprim-sulfamethoxazole, tetracyclines, and rifabutin [58].

Duration of treatment for NTM infections is usually prolonged. The recommended treatment duration for NTM pulmonary infections with MAC and *M. kansasii* is at least 12 months from culture negativity [1]. For *M. abscessus*, it is recommended that either a shorter or longer treatment regimen be used for pulmonary infections, and expert consultation should be sought [1]. For extrapulmonary MAC with skin tissue and skeletal disease, duration of treatment is usually 6–12 months [6]. Disseminated MAC infections in patients with advanced HIV may be able to stop MAC treatment after at least 12 months of therapy and with sustained CD4 counts >100 for at least 6 months [1]. Patients with disseminated *M. chimaera* after cardiac surgery were treated for 12 months and some more than 24 months [1, 39]. Catheter-related bacteremia is managed with removal of the catheter and therapy for 2 months after catheter removal [18]. For *M. abscessus*, *M. chelonae*, and *M. fortuitum* serious skin and soft tissue infections, a minimum of 4 months is recommended and 6 months for bone infections [6]. For patients with persistently positive cultures after 6 months of appropriate therapy, antimicrobial susceptibility testing should be repeated, and periodic testing of susceptibilities is useful in monitoring for emergence of drug resistance [50]. Therapeutic drug monitoring, such as for clarithromycin or azithromycin, can be considered in treatment failures, particularly in patients with absorption issues [59].

The use of multiple medications of prolonged duration to treat NTM infections means more drug side effects and toxicities. Adverse effects can lead to dose reductions, dose discontinuations, or treatment interruptions [48]. Patients should be monitored closely for side effects, with review of symptoms and laboratory monitoring (such as complete blood count, liver tests, creatinine, and in some cases, EKG monitoring). Drug-drug interactions should also be taken into account, particularly with rifampin. Use of ethambutol requires monitoring for vision changes as ethambutol can cause decreased visual acuity (optic neuritis) and can also cause peripheral neuropathy [40]. Side effects from azithromycin and clarithromycin include diarrhea, nausea, abdominal pain, hearing loss, elevated liver tests, and QT prolongation [40]. Rifampin and rifabutin use can lead to red/orange discoloration of secretions, hepatitis, and GI issues, as well as uveitis from rifabutin [60]. Rifamycins also cause flu-like syndrome and leukopenia and thrombocytopenia [40]. Parenteral amikacin is known to cause nephrotoxicity and ototoxicity, while dysphonia and respiratory symptoms such as dyspnea have been reported with inhaled amikacin [60]. Doxycycline can cause GI side effects and photosensitivity [60]. Fluoroquinolones also have multiple side effects such as GI symptoms (nausea, vomiting, abdominal pain), CNS effects (delirium, dizziness, insomnia), rash, transaminitis, tendonitis/rupture, and QT prolongation [40]. Clofazimine can cause dose-related hypergpigmentation of body tissues, skin dryness, photosensitivity, and GI side effects from crystal deposition [61]. Myelosuppression, lactic acidosis, and ocular and peripheral neuropathy have been described with linezolid [61]. Adverse effects of imipenem and cefoxitin include GI symptoms, cytopenias, and rash [60, 61]. Tigecycline can cause GI adverse effects, photosensitivity, hepatitis, and pancreatitis [61].

With NTM ocular infections, delay in diagnosis or initial misdiagnosis due to difficulty in identifying the infection leads to delay in treatment [62]. Approximately 61% of infections were diagnosed within 4 weeks of presentation in the retrospective study conducted by Girgis et al. [11]. NTM infection should be suspected in patients with an indolent course and delayed presentation after intervention [62]. Antibiotic therapy for NTM ophthalmic infections is based on sensitivity data and the clinical experience from therapy of non-ocular infections [10]. Due to variability in susceptibilities to macrolides and fluoroquinolones, antibiotic susceptibility testing should be performed on ocular isolates [18]. Aminoglycosides and quinolones are used in treatment of these ocular infections, typically through local instillations [50]. Successful treatment has been described using topical therapy (with antimicrobials such as clarithromycin, amikacin, and tobramycin) combined with ophthalmic solutions and quinolones [50]. Topical linezolid has also been used [18]. Successful treatment also requires surgical debridement of abscesses in tissues such as periorbital skin, orbital fat, and cornea [10]. For infections such as conjunctivitis, scleritis, keratitis, and possibly endophthalmitis, topical antibiotics are useful while systemic antibiotics are required for almost all NTM ocular and adnexal infections [10]. NTM eye infections require prolonged therapy with two or more active agents as these infections are clinically refractory and can recur after stopping treatment [10]. Aggressive surgical debridement with pars plana vitrectomy and repeated intravitreal antibiotic injections along with parenteral multidrug regimen for endogenous and postoperative NTM endophthalmitis is needed for infection eradication [10]. In a cluster of NTM endophthalmitis following cataract surgery by Hsu et al., the patients had very poor visual outcome despite aggressive treatment with pars plana vitrectomy and intravitreal injections of amikacin, IOL-capsule complex removal, and systemic antibiotic use (clarithromycin, tigecycline, and intravenous amikacin) [14]. Shah et al. reported frequent removal of ocular device in patients with NTM endophthalmitis [7]. For NTM buckle infections, surgical removal of buckle material was important in clearing the infection in the study by Chu et al. in Taiwan [19]. Kheir et al. reviewed 174 case reports on NTM and found that receipt of steroids prior to diagnosis of NTM ocular infection was more likely to have lack of initial resolution to medical therapy, was more likely to have prolonged course of infection, and was less likely to have resolution of infection [62].

Unlike in other manifestations of NTM ocular infections, which were frequently associated with poor outcomes, patients with isolated *M. chimaera* chorioretinitis generally maintained good vision in the range of 20/20 to 20/25. This favorable ophthalmic outcome occurred despite lengthy delays from the time of cardiac surgery and infection to the time of ophthalmic diagnosis (median time 25 months) [17]. The lack of ophthalmic symptoms and good visual outcome associated with *M. chimaera* choroiditis are also in contrast to the systemic disease course, which was often severe or fatal due to the recalcitrant nature of the infection.

Case Report

A 65-year-old man with a history of aortic valve replacement (AVR), right rotator cuff repair, and bronchitis was seen in the eye clinic as part of an inpatient infectious work-up for low-grade fever of unknown origin (FUO). Fourteen months prior to presentation in the eye clinic, the patient underwent uncomplicated AVR via median sternotomy for a bicuspid aortic valve with severe aortic stenosis. Two months before presentation, the patient had undergone arthroscopy of the right shoulder and right rotator cuff repair. Shortly thereafter the patient developed persistent low-grade fever, malaise, and night sweats. The patient's medications included warfarin, aspirin, metoprolol, amlodipine, and atorvastatin. He did not smoke cigarettes, drink alcohol, or use other illicit drugs. He had no significant past ocular history, and at the time of evaluation he did not have any eye or visual complaints.

On examination, BCVA was 20/20 in both eyes, and intraocular pressures (IOP) were 11 mmHg in both eyes. There was no afferent pupillary defect, and the anterior chambers of both eyes were normal. On dilated fundus exam, however, there were creamy-yellow subretinal infiltrates distributed throughout the posterior pole and mid-periphery in both eyes. FA demonstrated staining of the subretinal lesions and vascular leakage peripherally. ICGA revealed punctate areas of blockage more numerous than the lesions seen on exam or FA (Fig. 2.1a–f). An infectious and inflammatory work-up was initiated, and tests results for tuberculosis, syphilis, *Bartonella*, *Legionella*, and CMV were negative. Blood cultures were obtained during his hospital admission but remained negative at the time of his discharge 1 week later. A chest computed tomography scan and a liver biopsy both suggested granulomatous inflammation, prompting concern for sarcoidosis. He was started on high-dose prednisone, and choroidal lesions were observed to improve over 3 weeks.

Thirty-three days after initially being drawn, blood cultures became positive for acid-fast bacilli which were subsequently identified as *M. chimaera* based on 16S ribosomal DNA sequencing. Repeat cultures were similarly positive. The patient was started on rifabutin, ethambutol, and azithromycin and has remained on these antibiotics through the subsequent 18 months of follow-up. Throughout this follow-up period, the patient continued to have 20/20 BCVA in both eyes; choroidal lesions improved with treatment but did not resolve completely (Fig. 2.1g, h), and new lesions could be seen with continued systemic infection. He subsequently underwent two additional AVR reoperations but continued to have persistence of systemic infection afterwards.

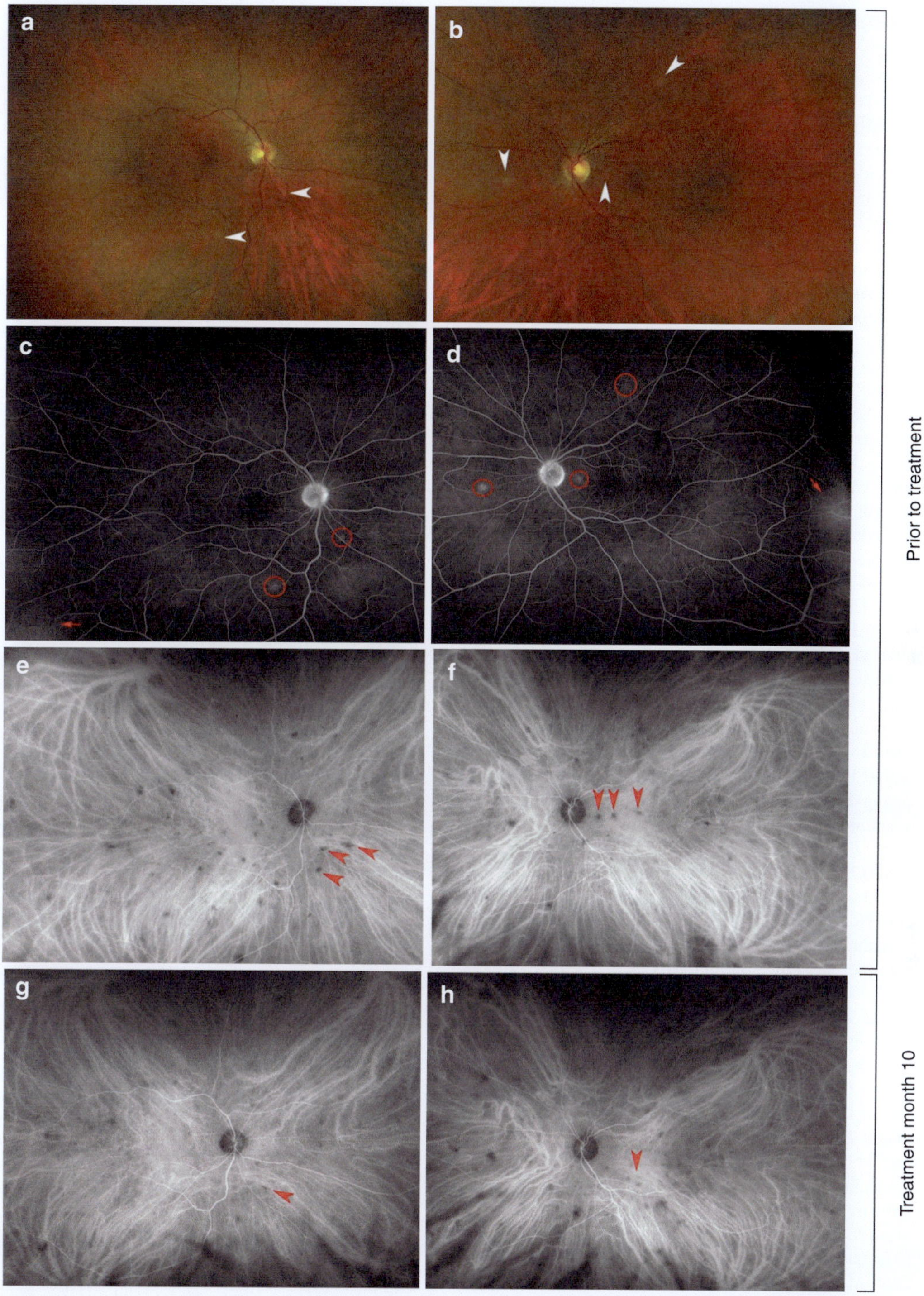

Fig. 2.1 Multimodal ophthalmic imaging in a patient with *M. chimaera* multifocal choroiditis. (**a**, **b**) A few small, yellow-white choroidal lesions could be seen in both eyes distributed throughout the posterior pole and mid-periphery (white arrowheads). (**c**, **d**) These lesions correlated with areas of staining on FA (red circles). A few areas of peripheral vascular leakage (red arrows) could also be seen in both eyes. (**e**, **f**) Lesions could also be seen on ICGA (red arrowheads) and were relatively more numerous than what could be seen on fundus exam or FA. (**g**, **h**) With treatment, lesions can resolve on exam and imaging, but with continued infection new lesions will appear as can be seen in follow-up ICGA 10 months after initiation of treatment

References

1. Daley CL. Treatment of nontuberculous mycobacterial pulmonary disease: an official ATS/ERS/ESCMID/IDSA clinical practice guideline. Eur Respir J. 2020;56
2. Koh W-J. Nontuberculous Mycobacteria—overview. Microbiol Spectr. 2017:5. https://doi.org/10.1128/microbiolspec.TNMI7-0024-2016.
3. Falkinham JO. Nontuberculous mycobacteria from household plumbing of patients with nontuberculous mycobacteria disease. Emerg Infect Dis. 2011;17:419–24. https://doi.org/10.3201/eid1703.101510.
4. Honda JR, Knight V, Chan ED. Pathogenesis and risk factors for nontuberculous mycobacterial lung disease. Clin Chest Med. 2015;36:1–11. https://doi.org/10.1016/j.ccm.2014.10.001.
5. Falkinham JO. Challenges of NTM drug development. Front Microbiol. 2018;9:1613. https://doi.org/10.3389/fmicb.2018.01613.
6. Griffith DE, Aksamit T, Brown-Elliott BA, Catanzaro A, Daley C, Gordin F, et al. An official ATS/IDSA statement: diagnosis, treatment, and prevention of nontuberculous mycobacterial diseases. Am J Respir Crit Care Med. 2007;175:367–416. https://doi.org/10.1164/rccm.200604-571ST.
7. Shah M, Relhan N, Kuriyan AE, Davis JL, Albini TA, Pathengay A, et al. Endophthalmitis caused by nontuberculous mycobacterium: clinical features, antimicrobial susceptibilities, and treatment outcomes. Am J Ophthalmol. 2016;168:150–6. https://doi.org/10.1016/j.ajo.2016.03.035.
8. Huang SC, Soong HK, Chang JS, Liang YS. Nontuberculous mycobacterial keratitis: a study of 22 cases. Br J Ophthalmol. 1996;80:962–8. https://doi.org/10.1136/bjo.80.11.962.
9. Chandra NS, Torres MF, Winthrop KL, Bruckner DA, Heidemann DG, Calvet HM, et al. Cluster of Mycobacterium Chelonae keratitis cases following laser in-situ keratomileusis. Am J Ophthalmol. 2001;132:819–30. https://doi.org/10.1016/S0002-9394(01)01267-3.
10. Moorthy RS, Valluri S, Rao NA. Nontuberculous mycobacterial ocular and adnexal infections. Surv Ophthalmol. 2012;57:202–35. https://doi.org/10.1016/j.survophthal.2011.10.006.
11. Girgis DO, Karp CL, Miller D. Ocular infections caused by non-tuberculous mycobacteria: update on epidemiology and management: ocular mycobacterial infections. Clin Exp Ophthalmol. 2012;40:467–75. https://doi.org/10.1111/j.1442-9071.2011.02679.x.
12. Holland SP, Pulido JS, Miller D, Ellis B, Alfonso E, Scott M, et al. Biofilm and scleral buckle-associated infections. Ophthalmology. 1991;98:933–8. https://doi.org/10.1016/S0161-6420(91)32199-7.
13. Chang V, Karp CL, Yoo SH, Ide T, Budenz DL, Kovach JL, et al. Mycobacterium abscessus endophthalmitis after Descemet's stripping with automated endothelial keratoplasty. Cornea. 2010;29:586–9. https://doi.org/10.1097/ICO.0b013e3181bd44b4.
14. Hsu C-R, Chen J-T, Yeh K-M, Hsu C-K, Tai M-C, Chen Y-J, et al. A cluster of nontuberculous mycobacterial endophthalmitis (NTME) cases after cataract surgery: clinical features and treatment outcomes. Eye. 2018;32:1504–11. https://doi.org/10.1038/s41433-018-0108-1.
15. Ambler JS, Meisler DM, Zakov ZN, Hall GS, Spech TJ. Endogenous mycobacterium chelonae endophthalmitis. Am J Ophthalmol. 1989;108:338–9. https://doi.org/10.1016/0002-9394(89)90136-0.
16. Williamson D, Howden B, Stinear T. *Mycobacterium chimaera* spread from heating and cooling units in heart surgery. N Engl J Med. 2017;376:600–2. https://doi.org/10.1056/NEJMc1612023.
17. Zweifel SA, Mihic-Probst D, Curcio CA, Barthelmes D, Thielken A, Keller PM, et al. Clinical and histopathologic ocular findings in disseminated Mycobacterium chimaera infection after cardiothoracic surgery. Ophthalmology. 2017;124:178–88. https://doi.org/10.1016/j.ophtha.2016.09.032.
18. Holt M, Kasperbauer S. Management of extrapulmonary nontuberculous mycobacterial infections. Semin Respir Crit Care Med. 2018;39:399–410. https://doi.org/10.1055/s-0038-1651490.
19. Chu H-S, Chang S-C, Shen EP, Hu F-R. Nontuberculous mycobacterial ocular infections—comparing the clinical and microbiological characteristics between mycobacterium abscessus and Mycobacterium massiliense. PLoS One. 2015;10:e0116236. https://doi.org/10.1371/journal.pone.0116236.
20. Mauriello JA, Atypical Mycobacterial Study Group. Atypical mycobacterial infection of the periocular region after periocular and facial surgery. Ophthal Plast Reconstr Surg. 2003;19:182–8. https://doi.org/10.1097/01.iop.0000064994.09803.cb.
21. Oz O, Lee DH, Smetana SM, Akduman L. A case of infected scleral buckle with mycobacterium chelonae associated with chronic intraocular inflammation. Ocul Immunol Inflamm. 2004;12:65–7. https://doi.org/10.1076/ocii.12.1.65.28069.
22. Pope J, Sternberg P, McLane NJ, Potts DW, Stulting RD. Mycobacterium chelonae scleral abscess after removal of a scleral buckle. Am J Ophthalmol. 1989;107:557–8. https://doi.org/10.1016/0002-9394(89)90511-4.
23. Margo CE. Mycobacterium chelonae conjunctivitis and scleritis following vitrectomy. Arch Ophthalmol. 2000;118:1125. https://doi.org/10.1001/archopht.118.8.1125.
24. Smiddy WE, Miller D, Flynn HW. Scleral buckle infections due to atypical mycobacteria. Retina. 1991;11:394–8. https://doi.org/10.1097/00006982-199111040-00005.
25. Sossi N. Mycobacterium gordonae keratitis after penetrating keratoplasty. Arch Ophthalmol.

1991;109:1064. https://doi.org/10.1001/archopht.1991.01080080022011.
26. Lalitha P, Rathinam SR, Srinivasan M. Ocular infections due to non-tuberculous mycobacteria. Indian J Med Microbiol. 2004;22(4):231–7. https://pubmed-ncbi-nlm-nih-gov.ccmain.ohionet.org/17642744/.
27. Matieli LCV, De Freitas D, Sampaio J, Moraes NSB, Yu MCZ, Hofling-Lima AL. Mycobacterium abscessus endophthalmitis: treatment dilemma and review of the literature. Retina. 2006;26:826–9. https://doi.org/10.1097/01.iae.0000244276.80716.96.
28. Ramaswamy A. Postoperative mycobacterium chelonae endophthalmitis after extracapsular cataract extraction and posterior chamber intraocular lens implantation. Ophthalmology. 2000;107:1283–6. https://doi.org/10.1016/S0161-6420(00)00162-7.
29. Roussel TJ, Stern WH, Goodman DF, Whitcher JP. Postoperative mycobacterial endophthalmitis. Am J Ophthalmol. 1989;107:403–6. https://doi.org/10.1016/0002-9394(89)90664-8.
30. Cohen JI, Saragas SJ. Endophthalmitis due to Mycobacterium avium in a patient with AIDS. Ann Ophthalmol. 1990;22:47–51.
31. Rosenbaum PS. Atypical mycobacterial panophthalmitis seen with iris nodules. Arch Ophthalmol. 1998;116:1524. https://doi.org/10.1001/archopht.116.11.1524.
32. Morinelli EN, Dugel PU, Riffenburgh R, Rao NA. Infectious multifocal choroiditis in patients with acquired immune deficiency syndrome. Ophthalmology. 1993;100:1014–21. https://doi.org/10.1016/S0161-6420(93)31543-5.
33. Wassermann HE. Avian tuberculosis endophthalmitis. Arch Ophthalmol. 1973;89:321–3. https://doi.org/10.1001/archopht.1973.01000040323013.
34. Bhikoo R, Bevan R, Sims J. Multifocal choroiditis with panuveitis in a patient with disseminated mycobacterium avium complex. Retin Cases Brief Rep. 2013;7:155–7. https://doi.org/10.1097/ICB.0b013e3182790ef9.
35. Kuznetcova TI, Sauty A, Herbort CP. Uveitis with occult choroiditis due to mycobacterium kansasii: limitations of interferon-gamma release assay (IGRA) tests (case report and mini-review on ocular non-tuberculous mycobacteria and IGRA cross-reactivity). Int Ophthalmol. 2012;32:499–506. https://doi.org/10.1007/s10792-012-9588-3.
36. Böni C, Al-Sheikh M, Hasse B, Eberhard R, Kohler P, Hasler P, et al. Multimodal imaging of choroidal lesions in disseminated mycobacterium chimaera infection after cardiothoracic surgery. Retina. 2019;39:452–64. https://doi.org/10.1097/IAE.0000000000001991.
37. Scriven JE, Scobie A, Verlander NQ, Houston A, Collyns T, Cajic V, et al. Mycobacterium chimaera infection following cardiac surgery in the United Kingdom: clinical features and outcome of the first 30 cases. Clin Microbiol Infect. 2018;24:1164–70. https://doi.org/10.1016/j.cmi.2018.04.027.
38. Lau D, Cooper R, Chen J, Sim VL, McCombe JA, Tyrrell GJ, et al. Mycobacterium chimaera encephalitis following cardiac surgery: a new syndrome. Clin Infect Dis. 2019:ciz497. https://doi.org/10.1093/cid/ciz497.
39. Kasperbauer SH, Daley CL. Mycobacterium chimaera infections related to the Heater–Cooler unit outbreak: a guide to diagnosis and management. Clin Infect Dis. 2019;68:1244–50. https://doi.org/10.1093/cid/ciy789.
40. Daley CL. Mycobacterium avium complex disease. Microbiol Spectr. 2017:5. https://doi.org/10.1128/microbiolspec.TNMI7-0045-2017.
41. Winthrop KL, Marras TK, Adjemian J, Zhang H, Wang P, Zhang Q. Incidence and prevalence of non-tuberculous mycobacterial lung disease in a large U.S. managed care health plan, 2008–2015. Ann Am Thorac Soc. 2020;17:178–85. https://doi.org/10.1513/AnnalsATS.201804-236OC.
42. van Ingen J. Microbiological diagnosis of non-tuberculous mycobacterial pulmonary disease. Clin Chest Med. 2015;36:43–54. https://doi.org/10.1016/j.ccm.2014.11.005.
43. Brown-Elliott BA, Philley JV. Rapidly growing mycobacteria. Microbiol Spectr. 2017:5. https://doi.org/10.1128/microbiolspec.TNMI7-0027-2016.
44. Duarte RS, Lourenco MCS, Fonseca LDS, Leao SC, Amorim EDLT, Rocha ILL, et al. Epidemic of post-surgical infections caused by Mycobacterium massiliense. J Clin Microbiol. 2009;47:2149–55. https://doi.org/10.1128/JCM.00027-09.
45. Schnabel D, Gaines J, Nguyen DB, Esposito DH, Ridpath A, Yacisin K, et al. Rapidly growing nontuberculous mycobacterium wound infections among medical tourists undergoing cosmetic surgeries in the Dominican Republic—Multiple States, March 2013–February 2014. MMWR Morb Mortal Wkly Rep. 2014;63:201–2.
46. Perkins KM, Lawsin A, Hasan NA, Strong M, Halpin AL, Rodger RR, et al. *Notes from the field* : *Mycobacterium chimaera* contamination of heater-cooler devices used in cardiac surgery — United States. MMWR Morb Mortal Wkly Rep. 2016;65:1117–8. https://doi.org/10.15585/mmwr.mm6540a6.
47. Asadi T, Mullin K, Roselli E, Johnston D, Tan CD, Rodriguez ER, et al. Disseminated Mycobacterium chimaera infection associated with heater–cooler units after aortic valve surgery without endocarditis. J Thorac Cardiovasc Surg. 2018;155:2369–74. https://doi.org/10.1016/j.jtcvs.2017.12.049.
48. Kasperbauer SH, De Groote MA. The treatment of rapidly growing mycobacterial infections. Clin Chest Med. 2015;36:67–78. https://doi.org/10.1016/j.ccm.2014.10.004.
49. van Ingen J. Diagnosis of nontuberculous mycobacterial infections. Semin Respir Crit Care Med. 2013;34:103–9. https://doi.org/10.1055/s-0033-1333569.

50. Brown-Elliott BA, Nash KA, Wallace RJ. Antimicrobial susceptibility testing, drug resistance mechanisms, and therapy of infections with nontuberculous mycobacteria. Clin Microbiol Rev. 2012;25:545–82. https://doi.org/10.1128/CMR.05030-11.
51. Brown-Elliott BA, Woods GL. Antimycobacterial susceptibility testing of nontuberculous mycobacteria. J Clin Microbiol. 2019;57:e00834–19., /jcm/57/10/JCM.00834-19.atom. https://doi.org/10.1128/JCM.00834-19.
52. Wang M-S, Wang J-L, Wang X-F. The performance of interferon-gamma release assay in nontuberculous mycobacterial diseases: a retrospective study in China. BMC Pulm Med. 2016;16:163. https://doi.org/10.1186/s12890-016-0320-3.
53. Busin M, Ponzin D, Arffa RC. Mycobacterium chelonae interface infection after endokeratoplasty. Am J Ophthalmol. 2003;135:393–5. https://doi.org/10.1016/S0002-9394(02)01954-2.
54. Stewart MW, Alvarez S, Ginsburg WW, Shetty R, McLain WC, Sleater JP. Visual recovery following *Mycobacterium chelonae* endophthalmitis. Ocul Immunol Inflamm. 2006;14:181–3. https://doi.org/10.1080/09273940600678062.
55. Greendyke R, Byrd TF. Differential antibiotic susceptibility of Mycobacterium abscessus variants in biofilms and macrophages compared to that of planktonic bacteria. Antimicrob Agents Chemother. 2008;52:2019–26. https://doi.org/10.1128/AAC.00986-07.
56. Lee SH, Yoo HK, Kim SH, Koh W-J, Kim CK, Park YK, et al. The drug resistance profile of *Mycobacterium abscessus* group strains from Korea. Ann Lab Med. 2014;34:31–7. https://doi.org/10.3343/alm.2014.34.1.31.
57. Griffith D. Treatment of Mycobacterium avium complex (MAC). Semin Respir Crit Care Med. 2018;39:351–61. https://doi.org/10.1055/s-0038-1660472.
58. Philley JV, Griffith DE. Treatment of slowly growing mycobacteria. Clin Chest Med. 2015;36:79–90. https://doi.org/10.1016/j.ccm.2014.10.005.
59. Peloquin C. The role of therapeutic drug monitoring in mycobacterial infections. Microbiol Spectr. 2017:5. https://doi.org/10.1128/microbiolspec.TNMI7-0029-2016.
60. Shulha JA, Escalante P, Wilson JW. Pharmacotherapy approaches in nontuberculous mycobacteria infections. Mayo Clin Proc. 2019;94:1567–81. https://doi.org/10.1016/j.mayocp.2018.12.011.
61. Egelund EF, Fennelly KP, Peloquin CA. Medications and monitoring in nontuberculous mycobacteria infections. Clin Chest Med. 2015;36:55–66. https://doi.org/10.1016/j.ccm.2014.11.001.
62. Kheir WJ, Sheheitli H, Abdul Fattah M, Hamam RN. Nontuberculous mycobacterial ocular infections: a systematic review of the literature. Biomed Res Int. 2015;2015:1–17. https://doi.org/10.1155/2015/164989.

3 Syphilis: Emerging Ocular Infections

Jessica L. Cao, Careen Y. Lowder, and Steven M. Gordon

Abbreviations

ASPPC	acute syphilitic posterior placoid chorioretinitis
CDC	Centers for Disease Control
CNS	central nervous system
CSF	cerebrospinal fluid
LP	lumbar puncture
MMWR	Morbidity and Mortality Weekly Report
MSM	men who have sex with men
MSW	men who have sex with women only
OCT	optical coherence tomography
OD	right eye
OS	left eye
OU	both eyes
P&S	primary and secondary
RPE	retinal pigment epithelium
RPR	rapid plasma reagin
STD	sexually transmitted disease
TP-EIA	*T. pallidum* enzyme immunoassay
USA	United States of America
VDRL	Venereal Disease Research Laboratory

J. L. Cao (✉)
Department of Ophthalmology, Cleveland Clinic, Cole Eye Institute, Cleveland, OH, USA

The Retina Partners, Los Angeles, California, USA

C. Y. Lowder
Department of Ophthalmology, Cleveland Clinic, Cole Eye Institute, Cleveland, OH, USA
e-mail: lowderc@ccf.org

S. M. Gordon
Department of Infectious Disease, Cleveland Clinic, Cleveland, OH, USA
e-mail: gordons@ccf.org

Introduction

In 2015, about 45.4 million people were infected with syphilis, and six million new cases were diagnosed globally [1]. In the United States, between 2013 and 2017, the national annual rate of reported primary and secondary (P&S) syphilis cases increased 72.7%, from 5.5 to 9.5 cases per 100,000 population [2]. The highest rates of P&S syphilis are seen among gay, bisexual, and other men who have sex with men (collectively referred to as MSM), and MSM continued to account for the majority of cases in 2017. However, between 2013 and 2017, the P&S syphilis rate among women increased 155.6% (from 0.9 to 2.3 cases per 100,000 women), and the rate among all men increased 65.7% (from 10.2 to 16.9 cases per 100,000 men), indicating increasing transmission between men and women in addition to increasing transmission between MSM. To further understand these trends, the Centers for Disease Control and Prevention (CDC) analyzed national P&S syphilis surveillance data between 2013 and 2017 and assessed the percentage of cases among women, men who have sex with women only (MSW), and MSM who reported drug-related risk behaviors during the prior 12 months. Among women and MSW with P&S syphilis, reported

© Springer Nature Switzerland AG 2023
C. Y. Lowder et al. (eds.), *Emerging Ocular Infections*, Essentials in Ophthalmology,
https://doi.org/10.1007/978-3-031-24559-6_3

use of methamphetamine, injection drugs, and heroin more than doubled between 2013 and 2017. In 2017, 16.6% of women with P&S syphilis used methamphetamine, 10.5% used injection drugs, and 5.8% used heroin during the preceding 12 months. Similar trends were seen among MSW, but not among MSM. These findings indicate that a substantial percentage of heterosexual syphilis transmission is occurring among persons who use these drugs, particularly methamphetamine. Collaboration between sexually transmitted disease (STD) control programs and partners that provide substance use disorder services will be important to address recent increases in heterosexual syphilis.

As rates of syphilis have risen, there has also been a corresponding rise in ocular syphilis. A recent article in Morbidity and Mortality Weekly Report (MMWR) detailed 12 cases of ocular syphilis from San Francisco and Seattle [3]. Because of concerns about an increase in ocular syphilis, eight jurisdictions (California [excluding Los Angeles and San Francisco], Florida, Indiana, Maryland, New York City, North Carolina, Texas, and Washington) reviewed syphilis surveillance and case investigation data from 2014, 2015, or both to ascertain syphilis cases with ocular manifestations. A total of 388 suspected ocular syphilis cases were identified, 157 in 2014 and 231 in 2015. Overall, among total syphilis surveillance cases in the jurisdictions evaluated, 0.53% in 2014 and 0.65% in 2015 indicated ocular symptoms. Five jurisdictions described an increase in suspected ocular syphilis cases in 2014 and 2015. The predominance of cases in men (93%), MSM, and percentage who are HIV-positive (51%) are consistent with the epidemiology of syphilis in the United States. It is important for clinicians to be aware of potential visual complications related to syphilis infections. Prompt identification of potential ocular syphilis, ophthalmologic evaluation, and appropriate treatment are critical to prevent or manage visual symptoms and sequelae of ocular blindness.

In this chapter, we review the pathogenesis of syphilis, including the mode of transmission in both acquired and congenital cases and the route of entry to the eye. We then discuss clinical features on systemic and ocular exams and review current guidelines for testing for syphilis. The remainder of the chapter focuses on management and provides two clinical case examples of ocular syphilis.

Pathogenesis

Syphilis is a sexually transmitted infection caused by the bacterium species *Treponema pallidum* (subspecies pallidum), a spiral-shaped, Gram-negative, highly mobile bacterium. Three other human diseases are caused by related Treponema pallidum subspecies, including yaws (subspecies pertenue), pinta (subspecies carateum), and bejel (subspecies endemicum). Humans are the only known natural reservoir for the subspecies pallidum [4]. The non-venereal treponematosis contrasts dramatically with syphilis, which most commonly is transmitted through sexual activity, but it may also be transmitted from mother to baby during pregnancy or at birth, resulting in congenital syphilis. The spirochete is able to pass through intact mucous membranes or compromised skin. Thus, it is transmissible by kissing near a lesion, as well as oral, vaginal, and anal sex. Syphilis can also be transmitted by blood products, but the risk is low due to strict screening protocols of donated blood in many countries. The risk of transmission from sharing needles appears limited. It is not generally possible to contract syphilis through toilet seats, daily activities, hot tubs, or sharing eating [5]. The incubation period between syphilis infection and development of ocular syphilis has not been widely studied, but one recent report in a cohort of HIV-positive Japanese patients found a median time of 11 months (range 2.5–45 months) between serologic diagnosis of syphilis and presentation with symptoms compatible with ocular syphilis [6]. The time of serologic diagnosis of syphilis was defined as the middle of two dates: (1) date when both rapid plasma reagin (RPR) titer was at least 1:8 and TPHA was positive in a patient previously syphilis-negative or date when RPR titer increased by fourfold if the patient was previously syphilis-positive and (2) the most recent date preceding (1) when (1) was not fulfilled. This same study reported that 87.5% of their eight cases developed ocular syphilis within 2 years of syphilis infection. It is postulated that HIV-infected persons may present with disease earlier and more frequently than those without HIV [7, 8].

Ocular syphilis is defined as laboratory-confirmed syphilis at any stage coupled with symptoms or signs of ocular disease consistent with syphilis. It may occur at any stage of infection, though it has been reported to be more common in secondary, tertiary, or latent stages and, in some cases, may even be the only clinical sign of syphilis [9]. In newly infected adults, the spirochete *Treponema pallidum* spreads through the bloodstream by penetrating endothelial tight junctions. It may also spread through lymphatics and ultimately invade the central nervous system (CNS) and its corresponding cerebrospinal fluid (CSF). This may result in ocular syphilis, which is considered a form of neurosyphilis as the eye is an extension of the CNS. Despite this, not all cases of ocular syphilis are accompanied by a syphilis-positive lumbar puncture (LP) or syphilitic meningitis [10]. It has been theorized that infection can later cause a destructive vasculitis involving ocular blood supply, leading to retinal or optic nerve ischemia [11]. Alternatively, it is possible that spirochetes directly invade the optic nerve head, leading to optic neuritis, or the optic-nerve sheath, causing optic perineuritis that leads to optic nerve atrophy [12]. In congenital cases, the fetus acquires the infection prior to birth from an infected mother. The spirochete is able to cross the placenta after about 14 weeks of gestation, after which it can disseminate and infect any fetal organ system [10].The fetus may also become infected if it contacts a syphilitic genital ulcer at the time of vaginal birth.

Clinical Features of Syphilis

The signs and symptoms of syphilis vary depending in which of the four stages it presents (primary, secondary, latent, and tertiary). The primary stage classically presents with a single chancre, a firm, painless, non-itchy skin ulceration usually between 1 and 2 cm in diameter, though there may be multiple sores. Primary syphilis is typically acquired by direct sexual contact with the infectious lesions of another person. Approximately 3–90 days after the initial exposure (average 21 days), a chancre appears at the point of contact. In 40% of cases, this is classically a single, firm, painless, non-itchy skin ulceration with a clean base and sharp borders approximately 0.3–3.0 cm in size [5]. In the classic form, it evolves from a macule to a papule and finally to an erosion or ulcer. The most common location is the cervix in women (44%), the penis in heterosexual men (99%), and anally and rectally in MSM (34%). Lymph node enlargement frequently (80%) occurs around the area of infection occurring 7 to 10 days after chancre formation. The lesion may persist for 3–6 weeks if left untreated [13].

Secondary syphilis occurs approximately 4–10 weeks after the primary infection and can involve the skin, mucous membranes, and lymph nodes. In secondary syphilis, a diffuse bodily rash consisting of reddish papules and nodules may develop (Fig. 3.1). The rash is non-itchy, generally symmetrical, reddish-pink, and characteristically on the palms and soles of feet [14].

Over time, the rash may become maculopapular or pustular. It may form flat, broad, whitish, wart-like lesions on mucous membranes, known as condyloma latum. In secondary syphilis, there may also be sores on mucosal surfaces in the mouth or vagina. All of these lesions harbor bacteria and are infectious. Systemic symptoms may

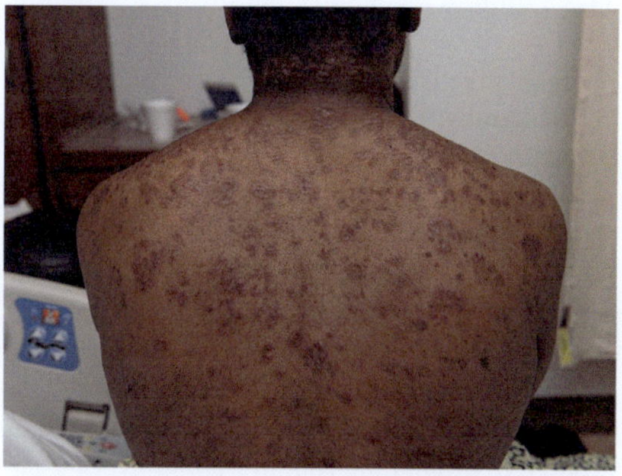

Fig. 3.1 Diffuse bodily rash consisting of reddish papules and nodules as seen in secondary syphilis

include fever, sore throat, malaise, weight loss, hair loss, and headache. Many people who present with secondary syphilis (40%–85% of women, 20–65% of men) do not report previously having had the classical chancre of primary syphilis [15].

In latent syphilis, which can last for years, there are few or no symptoms. Latent syphilis is defined as having serologic proof of infection without symptoms of disease. It is further described as either early (less than 1 year after secondary syphilis) or late (more than 1 year after secondary syphilis) in the United States. Early latent syphilis may have a relapse of symptoms. Late latent syphilis is asymptomatic and not as contagious as early latent syphilis [16].

In tertiary syphilis, there are gummas (soft, non-cancerous growths), neurological problems, or heart symptoms. Tertiary syphilis may occur approximately 3–15 years after the initial infection and may be divided into three different forms: gummatous syphilis (15%), late neurosyphilis (6.5%), and cardiovascular syphilis (10%). People with tertiary syphilis are not infectious [16]. Neurosyphilis refers to an infection involving the CNS. In the United States, the prevalence of neurosyphilis was 1.8% among patients with early syphilis in ten states with regular case reporting [17]. It may occur early, being either asymptomatic early neurosyphilis or syphilitic meningitis, early or late as meningovascular syphilis, or late as general paresis or tabes dorsalis [17].

Late neurosyphilis typically occurs 4–25 years after the initial infection. Meningovascular syphilis is a form of meningitis that involves vasculitis of small and medium-sized arteries in the CNS and typically presents as stroke, cranial nerve palsies or meningomyelitis with progressive myelopathy with apathy and seizures, and general paresis with dementia and tabes dorsalis [18].

Patients with general paresis present with progressive dementia and psychiatric syndromes, with Argyll Robertson pupils in fewer than half of patients (bilateral small pupils that constrict when the person focuses on near objects (accommodation reflex) but do not constrict when exposed to bright light (pupillary reflex). Tabes is characterized by gait ataxia with Romberg's sign and in most cases by Argyll Robertson pupils and is rarer than general paresis [18].

Syphilis is known as "the great masquerader" or "the great mimicker" for its ability to affect essentially any ocular structure. Because it may present in many different ways, ocular syphilis may pose a diagnostic challenge. Ocular syphilis may present at any stage of syphilis, but the rate of eye involvement is reportedly to be 10% in the secondary stage and 2–5% in the tertiary stage [19, 20]. Though it may present in patients of all ages, it usually presents in the fifth decade of life [21, 22]. The age has been reported to be significantly higher in HIV-negative patients than in HIV-positive patients [21]. Ocular involvement may be unilateral or bilateral and granulomatous or non-granulomatous. Affected patients may be either immunocompetent or immunocompromised. Around 10% have permanent visual impairment [21, 23].

Clinical symptoms may include pain, flashing lights, redness, photophobia, blurry vision, and floaters. Ocular manifestations may vary based on the stage of disease. In patients with primary syphilis, patients may have eyelid chancres, epithelial or stromal keratitis, or a conjunctival chancre which usually presents as a nodule or papule with progressive induration.

During the secondary stage of syphilis, patients may present with periostitis of the orbit most often of the supraorbital rim and orbital roof, orbital myositis, dacryocystitis, episcleritis or diffuse or nodular scleritis, annular rashes of the eyelid skin, conjunctival mucous patches, or marginal corneal infiltrates. Anterior uveitis may be granulomatous or nongranulomatous and may include a hyphema or hypopyon. Iris papules or nodules may also develop. Posterior involvement manifests as vitritis, neuroretinitis, optic neuritis, optic perineuritis, yellow choroidal infiltrates, chorioretinitis, retinal vasculitis, and exudative retinal detachments. Cranial nerve palsies of the third, fourth, and sixth cranial nerves as well as visual field defects may also be seen.

Manifestations seen in the tertiary stage of syphilis include gummatous orbital inflammation which can lead to an orbital pseudotumor-like picture, superior orbital fissure syndrome, orbital apex syndrome with disc edema, and extraocular muscle palsies. Other manifestations may be present and include dacryoadenitis, non-purulent dacryocystitis, subcutaneous gummas of the eye-

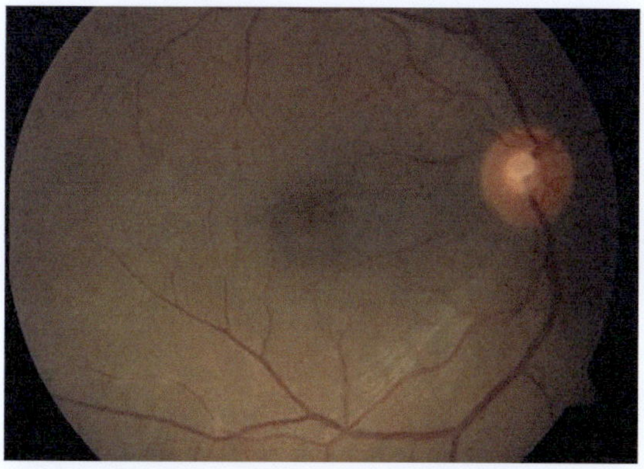

Fig. 3.2 Color fundus photo of a patient with ASPPC demonstrating faint large yellow placoid lesion within the macula

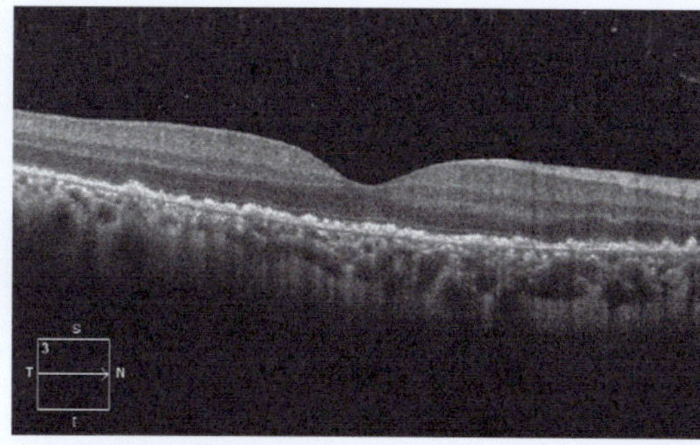

Fig. 3.3 OCT in ASPPC showing loss of the ellipsoid zone with dense hyperreflective granular material in the deep retina

lid, tarsitis, unilateral stromal keratitis with anterior uveitis, scleritis, anterior or posterior uveitis, granulomatous iris nodules, optic neuritis, optic perineuritis, and optic nerve gumma. Light-near dissociation in which the pupil constricts on near testing but does not constrict in response to light is another possible clinical feature.

There are three characteristic patterns of retinal manifestations, including acute syphilitic posterior placoid chorioretinitis (ASPPC), necrotizing retinitis, and punctate inner retinitis. In acute syphilitic posterior placoid chorioretinitis, fundus exam shows large gray to yellow placoid lesions involving the deep layers of the retina, including the retinal pigment epithelium (RPE) (Fig. 3.2). Lesions are typically in the macula and there is usually little inflammation. Optical coherence tomography (OCT) shows ellipsoid zone disruption with hyperreflective granular RPE changes and occasionally subretinal fluid (Fig. 3.3). After antibiotic treatment, the EZ layer and RPE may be reconstituted, though there may be persistent abnormalities. On fluorescein angiography, patients may have early hypofluorescent spots with late staining of placoid lesions (Fig. 3.4). Occasionally, there is punctate hypofluorescence known as "leopard spotting." On fundus autofluorescence, lesions are hyperautofluorescent, possibly due to outer retinal disruption unmasking the RPE fluorescence or lipofuscin accumulation at the level of the RPE-photoreceptor complex (Fig. 3.5). On

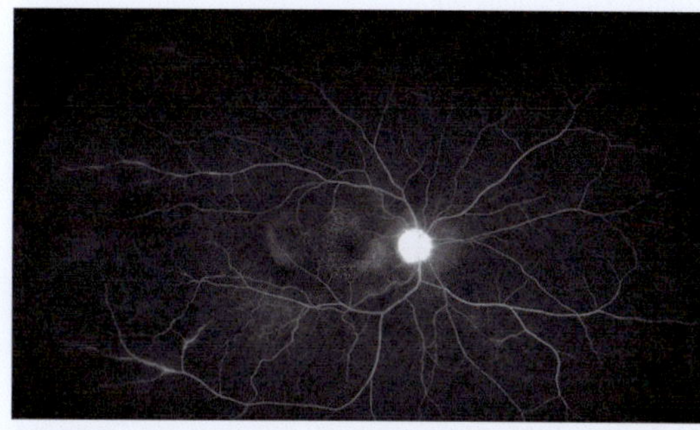

Fig. 3.4 Fluorescein angiography demonstrating hyperfluorescence of the placoid lesion within the macula in ASPPC. This image also shows punctate hypofluorescence, also known as "leopard spotting"

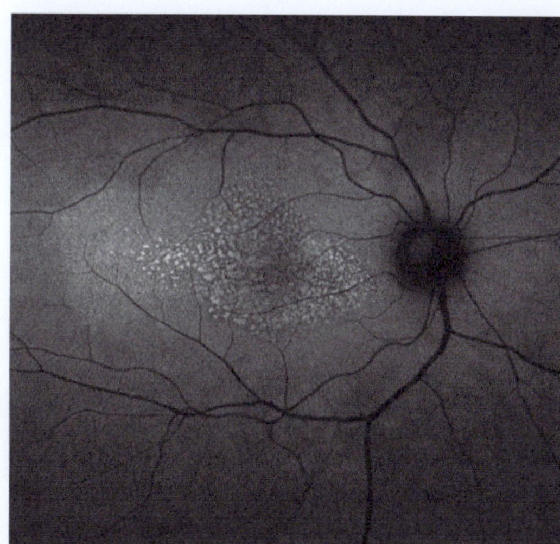

Fig. 3.5 Fundus autofluorescence showing hyperautofluorescence of placoid lesion in ASPPC

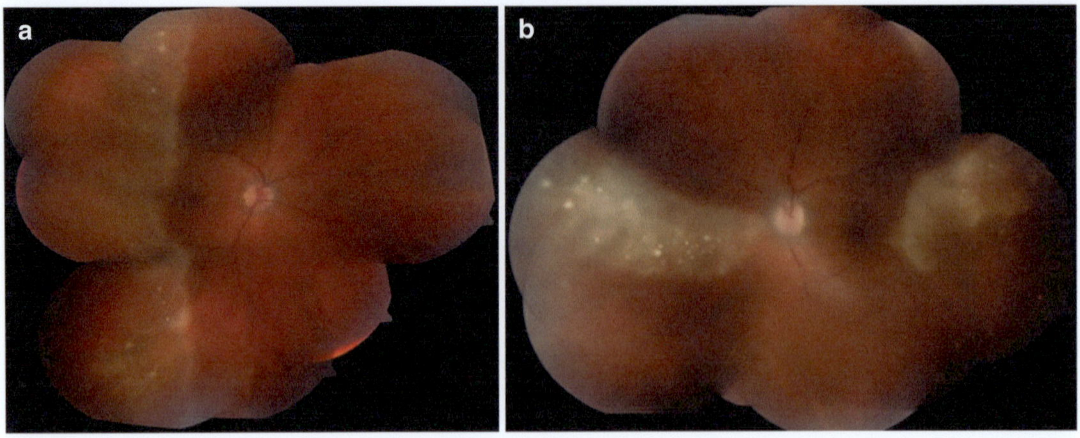

Fig. 3.6 (**a**) Fundus photo of inner retinal white punctate infiltrates and temporal arteriolar sheathing in punctate inner retinitis. (**b**) Fundus photo of inner retinal white punctate infiltrates in punctate inner retinitis

OCT angiography, patients may show reduced choriocapillaris flow [24].

In contrast, in necrotizing retinitis, the infection tends to involve the areas outside the arcades and mimics viral retinitis. There is retinal whitening on exam with prominent vitritis. In punctate inner retinitis, there are inner retinal and preretinal white infiltrates that may appear similar to "ground glass" (Fig. 3.6a, b). Patients may also have vitritis with sheathing of arterioles (see Fig. 3.6a). On OCT, there may be hyperreflectivity of the retina with dense focal hyperreflective intraretinal lesions. After the active phase of inflammation, there may be inner retinal atrophy with disruption of the ellipsoid zone and RPE [25].

Congenital syphilis manifestations may be subdivided into early and late stages. In the early stage, a chancre of the eyelid or papular skin rash of the lid, mucous patches of the conjunctiva or caruncle, iritis, multifocal choroiditis, or "salt-and-pepper" hypopigmented and hyperpigmented fundus spots may appear. In the late stage, cicatricial ectropions, eyelid gummas, anterior uveitis, chorioretinal scarring, or bilateral interstitial keratitis may be present. Interstitial keratitis usually presents as diffuse, ground-glass haziness deep within the cornea with superior stromal infiltrates and keratic precipitates. This progresses centrally and can coalesce or manifest as patchy multifocal infiltrates. Radial neovascularization with overlying inflammation appears red and is referred to as a "salmon patch." Interstitial keratitis, impaired hearing, and malformed teeth make up the "Hutchinson triad" characteristic of congenital syphilis. Signs of disease that can present in both stages include orbital periostitis, chronic dacryocystitis or dacryoadenitis, and congenital cataract.

Clinical outcomes may vary. A longer duration of uveitis before diagnosis or chorioretinitis in the macula at presentation may be associated with poorer vision [21]. Ocular syphilis is often accompanied with syphilitic meningitis, though this is not always the case. Lumbar puncture may be positive in only approximately half of patients [23]. HIV-positive patients are more likely to have abnormal lumbar punctures.

Laboratory Testing

Syphilis testing can be divided into two categories. Treponemal assays (syphilis IgG, TP IgG) measure antibodies that directly react with the syphilis-causing organism *T. pallidum*, while non-treponemal assays (RPR, VDRL [Venereal Disease Research Laboratory]) measure antibodies against non-specific cardiolipin antigens released during treponemal infections. In the traditional or classical testing algorithm for diagnosing syphilis, patient serum is initially tested with a non-treponemal test, followed by confirmation with a more specific treponemal test. This algorithm was popular because of the technical ease of performing the RPR relative to FTA or TP-EIA (*T. pallidum* enzyme immunoassay) testing. However, because the RPR test does not recognize treponemal-specific antibodies, a number of clinical situations could result in false-positive RPR results, including autoimmune disease, acute viral infection, recent immunizations, or persons who inject drugs. Most importantly, because RPR reactivity is a feature of active syphilis infection, the test could give false-negative results in latent or late syphilis. In 2015, the CDC began endorsing another testing algorithm (the reverse algorithm) in which the patient's blood is initially tested using a specific treponemal test and confirmed with a non-treponemal test. The reverse algorithm increases the yield for detecting patients with either very early syphilis or late syphilis. The RPR may be negative in these cases.

A reactive syphilis IgG result indicates that a person has been exposed to *T. pallidum* at some point in his/her life. However, this testing may remain reactive for life in the majority of people who have had syphilis, even if they have been treated properly. Therefore, a positive result does not indicate that the person currently has untreated syphilis, and the result should be confirmed with a non-treponemal test such as RPR to assess disease activity. If the follow-up non-treponemal test is reactive in the absence of a clinical history of treatment, it generally can be assumed that the patient has syphilis and should receive treatment. A positive RPR test is followed by a quantitative RPR with titer, which correlates with disease activity and can be used to monitor response to treatment. Most people become seronegative on non-treponemal tests following adequate treatment; however, some patients have a low RPR titer for life when they present with untreated late, latent, or tertiary disease, despite being adequately treated. These patients are referred to as being "serofast."

The Syphilis IgG test as the screening assay was recently replaced at the Cleveland Clinic by Syphilis Total (IgM + IgG) assay due to a recent change by the manufacturer to afford earlier serodiagnosis of syphilis. This is also in keeping with syphilis reverse testing sequence algorithm. The test principle (Multiplex Flow Immunoassay) and the platform (BioPlex® 2200, Bio-Rad) will remain the same; however, since this is a qualitative test, the index value will not be reported out, and there will be no weak positive category. The new syphilis testing algorithm is depicted in Fig. 3.7.

Limitations of the assay include the possibility of the "prozone effect," which may produce false-negative results on the RPR test due to excessively high antibody concentrations. In addition, when testing infants up to 15 months of age, those with reactive syphilis IgG and/or positive RPR should be tested for a positive IgM antibody as the infants will likely have had positive IgG antibodies from the mother.

Ocular syphilis is diagnosed when there is serologic evidence of syphilis coupled with ocular findings consistent with syphilitic infection. In all cases of ocular syphilis, a lumbar puncture (LP) should be performed as there is a high rate of neurosyphilis even in the absence of neurological symptoms. If the CSF is positive for VDRL, the LP should be repeated every 6 months until the cell count, protein, and VDRL have normalized. If the cell count has not decreased after 6 months, the clinician should consider retreatment [17].

Though vitreous sampling for nontreponemal and treponemal antibodies has been reported, direct sampling from the vitreous is not necessary if clinical presentation and serology are consistent with a diagnosis of syphilis [20]. In atypical cases, intraocular fluid sampling may be considered. PCR analysis of CSF, which is more specific, may also be considered in ambiguous cases. All patients who test positive for syphilis should undergo HIV testing as there is a high rate of co-infection. Clinicians should be aware that patients with HIV may have a higher rate of

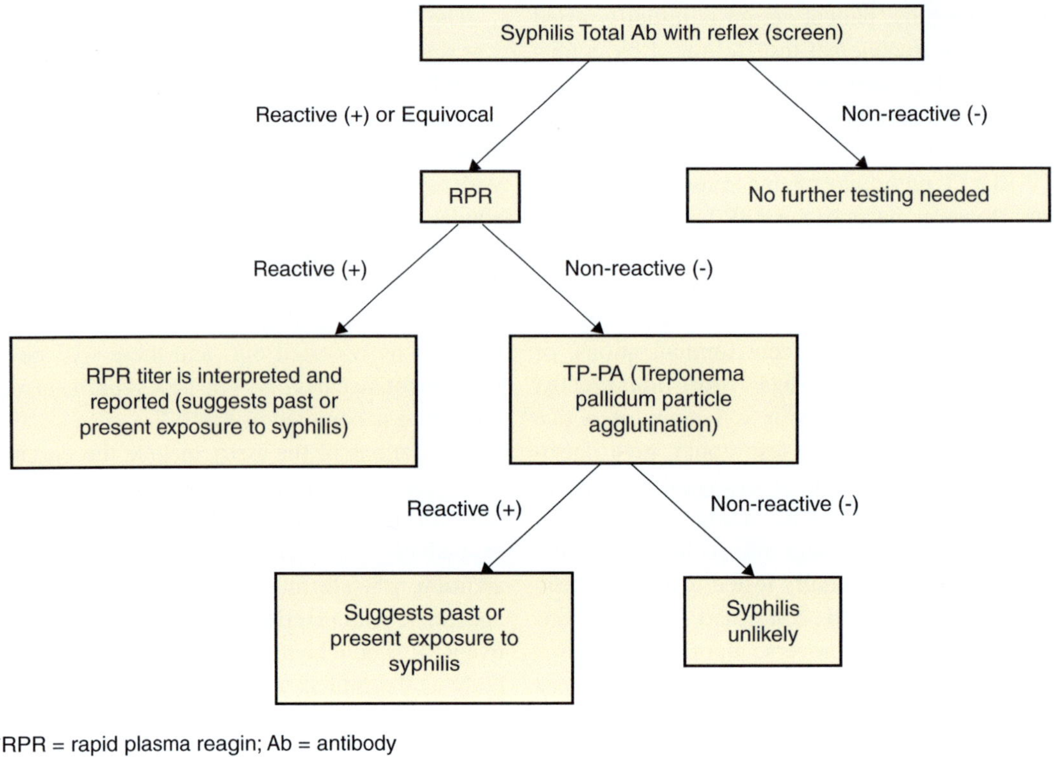

Fig. 3.7 Updated syphilis serology testing algorithm

false-negative and false-positive results on serology. False-positive results may also be possible in patients with autoimmune conditions, pregnancy, injection-drug use, advanced age, tuberculosis, vaccinations, malaria, atypical pneumonia, and Lyme disease.

Management

Syphilis can be effectively treated with antibiotics. The preferred antibiotic for most cases is benzathine benzylpenicillin injected into a muscle [26]. In those who have a severe penicillin allergy, doxycycline or tetracycline may be used if patients are not pregnant, coinfected with HIV, or diagnosed with neurosyphilis. In those with neurosyphilis, intravenous benzylpenicillin or ceftriaxone is recommended [26]. During treatment, patients may develop fever, headache, and muscle pains, an acute reaction known as Jarisch-Herxheimer. This reaction may occur within 24 hours of initiation of treatment and is an exaggerated host response due to bacteriolysis.

The main treatment for posterior segment ocular syphilis is identical to that of neurosyphilis, which includes penicillin G 18–24 million units/day given intravenously as 3 to 4 million U every 4 hours or continuously for 10–14 days. Alternatively, patients may receive 2.4 million units of intramuscular penicillin per day with oral probenecid 500 mg four times per day. Limited evidence suggests that ceftriaxone, tetracycline, or doxycycline is effective in the treatment of neurosyphilis [27].

Oral penicillin is not effective in the treatment of posterior segment ocular syphilis. Those with a penicillin allergy must be desensitized prior to treatment with penicillin. In addition to systemic penicillin, ophthalmologists can consider topical, periocular, and systemic steroids to help control intraocular inflammation. Once the patient has been appropriately treated with penicillin, steroids may be utilized without concurrent antibiotic treatment. Systemic penicillin is currently the mainstay of treatment, and there is currently no evidence for the use of intravitreal antibiotics.

Sexual partners should be notified of exposure and need for evaluation. If the patient is diagnosed with primary, secondary, or early latent syphilis, any partners with whom they have had sexual contact within the preceding 90 days prior to diagnosis should be treated presumptively even if serology is negative. Laboratory reporting of reactive syphilis testing is automatically reported to state and local health departments for public health interventions. If sexual contact was more than 90 days prior to diagnosis, they should be treated if test results are not immediately available or follow-up is uncertain. If testing is negative, the partner does not require treatment.

For infants aged 30 days or less, the recommended CDC treatment for congenital syphilis is aqueous crystalline penicillin 100,000 to 150,000 units/kg/day, administered as 50,000 units/kg/dose intravenously every 12 h for the first 7 days of life and every 8 h thereafter for a total of 10 days. An alternative regimen is procaine penicillin G 50,000 units/kg/dose as a single daily dose intramuscularly for 10 days [2]. If there is a penicillin allergy, the neonate should be desensitized prior to treatment with penicillin. If the infant or child is older than 30 days, the recommended regimen is aqueous crystalline penicillin G 200,000 to 300,000 units/kg/day intravenously, administered as 50,000 units/kg every 4 to 6 hours for a total of 10 days.

Cases

Case 1

A 49-year-old African-American man presented with bilateral blurry vision of 1 week duration. His best-corrected visual acuity was 20/250 in the right eye (OD) and 20/80 in the left eye (OS). His pupillary exam was unremarkable. Intraocular pressures were 10 mmHg OD and 21 mmHg OS. Confrontational visual fields and extraocular movements were normal in both eyes. Review of systems was positive only for night sweats. On slit-lamp exam, he had 1+ conjunctival injection in both eyes (OU), keratic precipitates OU, 2+ anterior chamber cell OU, and 2+ anterior vitreous cell OU. On dilated fundus exam, he had pigmentary changes in the macula, vascular sheathing, and peripheral retinal depigmentation, all in both eyes (Fig. 3.8a, b). OCT of the macula OU showed subretinal material at the level of the RPE in the macula with disruption of the ellipsoid zone (Fig. 3.9a, b). Fluorescein angiography OU showed stippled hyperfluorescent staining with punctate hypofluorescent spots within the macula with peripheral vascular leakage and optic nerve leakage (Fig. 3.10a, b).

The patient underwent serologic testing for syphilis, tuberculosis, and sarcoidosis. Syphilis IgG was positive with an RPR titer of 1:128. ACE was also elevated at 94, while TB testing was negative. Chest x-ray was unremarkable. CT chest showed subcentimeter nodular lesions;

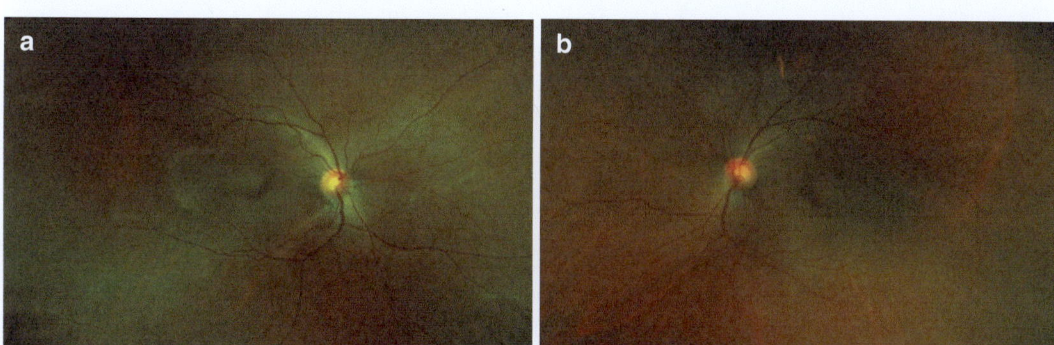

Fig. 3.8 (**a**) Fundus exam right eye showing pigmentary changes in macula. (**b**) Fundus exam left eye showing pigmentary changes in macula

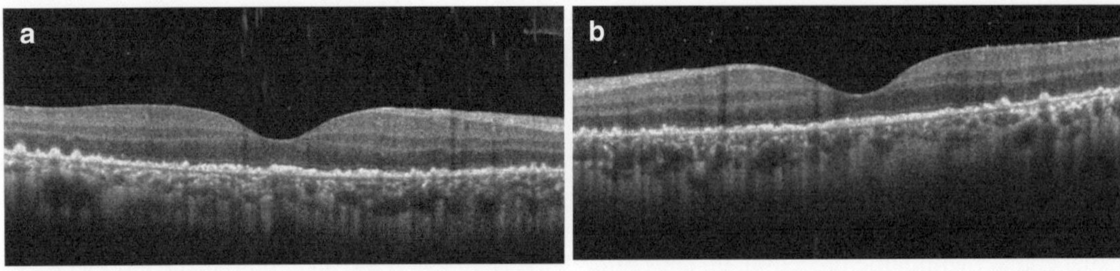

Fig. 3.9 (**a**, **b**) OCT of right eye (left image) and left eye (right image) showing deep subretinal hyperfluorescent lesions with profound disruption of the ellipsoid zone. Vitreous cell is apparent in both eyes in the posterior vitreous

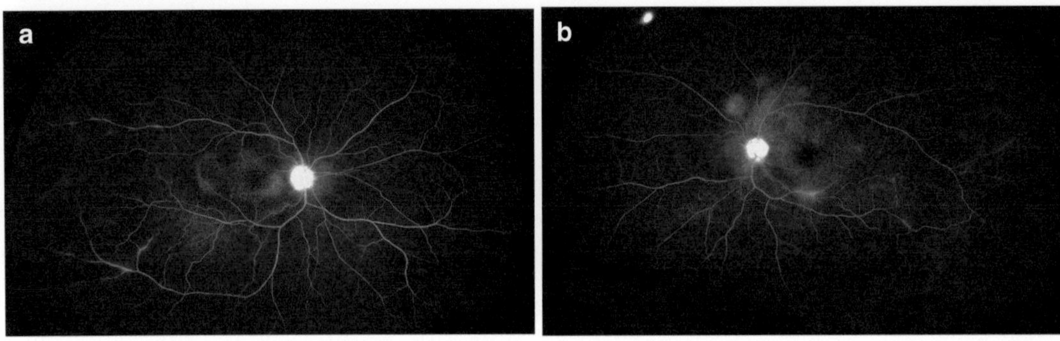

Fig. 3.10 (**a**, **b**) Stippled hyperfluorescent staining with punctate hypofluorescent spots within the macula with peripheral vascular leakage and optic nerve leakage in right and left eyes

however, biopsy of these lesions was not performed. Given concern for neurosyphilis, he was admitted to the hospital to start intravenous penicillin. He underwent an MRI of his brain and orbits with contrast, which was normal. Lumbar puncture showed unremarkable cell counts with negative CSF VDRL and FTA-Ab. He tested positive for HIV. He was started on intravenous penicillin G 4 million units every 4 h for 10 days.

On follow-up at the eye clinic 3 days later, vision had improved to 20/150 OD and was stable at 20/80 OS. The patient reported a subjective improvement in vision in both eyes. Given the presence of intraocular inflammation in the anterior chamber and vitreous, he was started on prednisolone acetate 1% topical drops four times daily in both eyes. Two days later, the inflammation had improved, but the fundus exam became suspicious for intraocular lymphoma given presence of "leopard spotting" (Fig. 3.11a, b).

Fortunately, CSF cytology was negative for lymphoma, and systemic CT imaging was unremarkable for lymphoma. Two days later, intraocular inflammation was improved with stable fluorescein angiography. OCT showed early reconstitution of the ellipsoid zone (Fig. 3.12a, b). Steroid eye drops were tapered down to twice a day, and he was started on oral prednisone 60 mg daily for persistent optic nerve leakage. When he returned 5 days later, vision had improved to 20/40 OD and 20/30 OS. Anterior chamber inflammation had resolved. His steroid eye drops and oral prednisone were both tapered. He returned 2 weeks later and was 20/20 OD and 20/25 OS. He was further tapered off his oral prednisone and was subsequently lost to follow-up.

Case 2

A 51-year-old African-American man was referred to the uveitis service for fluctuating blurry vision in both eyes over the last year. He

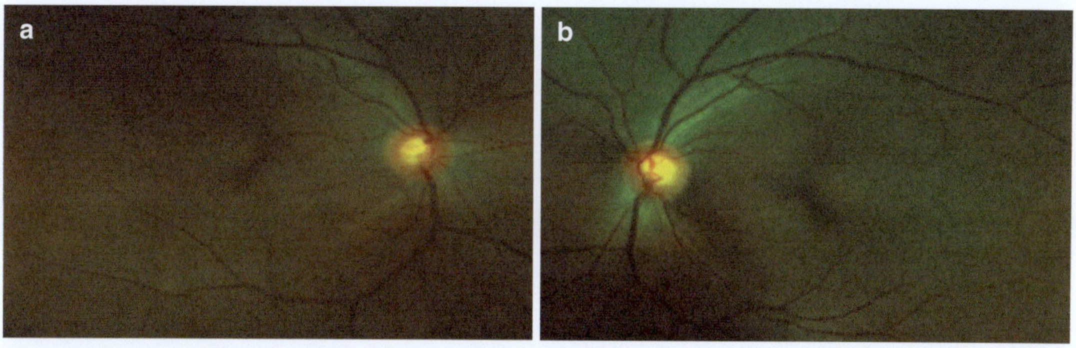

Fig. 3.11 (**a**, **b**) Stippled hypopigmented lesions of right and left eye, respectively, within the macula that appeared similar to "leopard spotting"

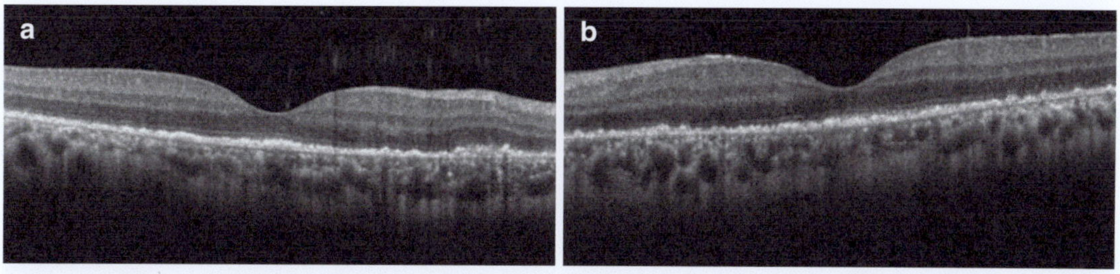

Fig. 3.12 (**a**, **b**) OCT of right and left eye, respectively, showing early reconstitution of ellipsoid zone

endorsed flashes and floaters as well as photophobia, worse in his left eye. Past medical and ocular history were non-contributory. He worked as a pastor and was married to a woman. He had a history of polysubstance abuse 2 years prior. On initial exam, vision was 20/100 OD and 20/60 OS. Intraocular pressures were 13 mmHg OD and 12 mmHg OS. Pupillary exam was unremarkable. On slit-lamp exam of the right eye, he had scattered keratic precipitates, 1+ AC cell, 2+ anterior vitreous cell, and haze. The left eye also had scattered keratic precipitates, 2+ AC cell, and 3+ anterior vitreous cell with snowballs. Dilated fundus exam showed slight optic nerve elevation, atrophy of the macula, vascular attenuation, and atrophy of the peripheral retina in both eyes (Fig. 3.13a, b). The OCTs of both eyes showed outer retinal loss, patchy disruption of the ellipsoid zone, and atrophy (Fig. 3.14a, b). Fluorescein angiography demonstrated diffuse vascular leakage and optic disc leakage in both eyes (Fig. 3.15a, b). He was started on prednisolone acetate 1% eye drops four times daily, and a work-up was pursued. Syphilis IgG was positive, and he had an RPR titer of 1:128. HIV testing was positive as well.

He subsequently was admitted to the hospital for management. He was evaluated by the Infectious Disease service and started IV penicillin 4 million units every 4 h for 2 weeks as well as HAART therapy for HIV. During his hospitalization, he underwent a lumbar puncture, which was positive for CSF VDRL. CT brain was normal. He was ultimately started on oral prednisone for management of intraocular inflammation. On his most recent follow-up, vision in the right eye was 20/50 and in the left eye, 20/25. A repeat RPR titer 3 months after treatment initiation was 1:64. His wife was tested and was fortunately negative for both HIV and syphilis.

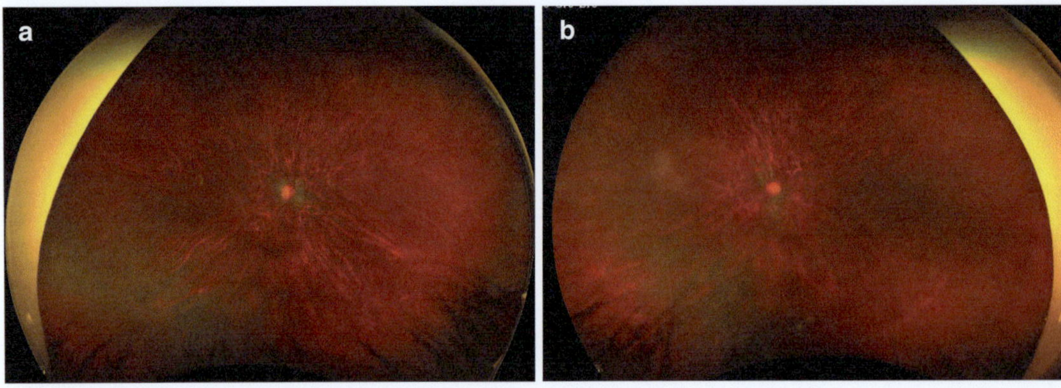

Fig. 3.13 (**a**, **b**) Optos fundus photos of the right and left eye, respectively

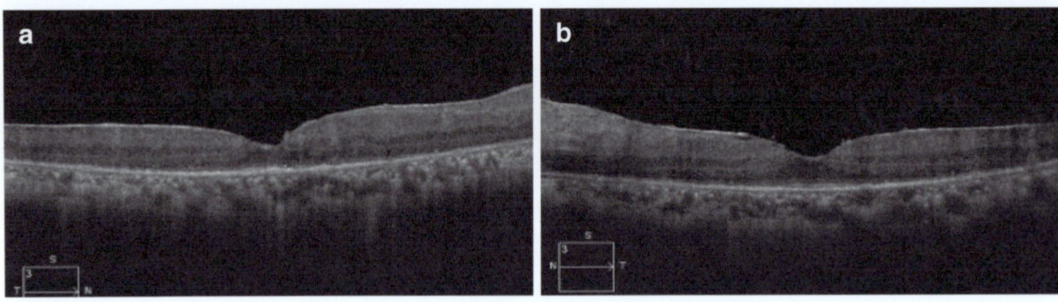

Fig. 3.14 (**a**, **b**) OCT of right and left eye, respectively, showing atrophy and significant ellipsoid zone loss

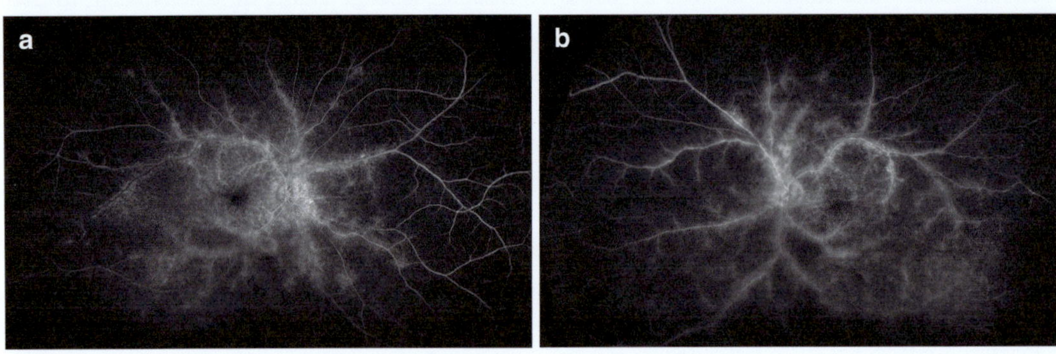

Fig. 3.15 (**a**, **b**) Fluorescein angiography of right and left eye, both showing diffuse vascular leakage and optic disc leakage

Summary

Ocular syphilis, a clinical manifestation of neurosyphilis, can involve almost any eye structure, but posterior uveitis and pan uveitis are the most common. Additional manifestations may include anterior uveitis, optic neuropathy, retinal vasculitis, and interstitial keratitis. Ocular syphilis may lead to decreased visual acuity including permanent blindness. While previous research supports evidence of neuropathogenic strains of syphilis, it remains unknown if some *Treponema pallidum* strains have a greater likelihood of causing ocular infections.

Clinicians should be aware of ocular syphilis and screen for visual complaints in any patient at risk for syphilis (MSM, HIV-infected persons, others with risk factors, and persons with multiple or anonymous partners). All patients with syphilis should receive an HIV test if status is unknown or previously HIV-negative. Patients with positive syphilis serology and early syphilis without ocular symptoms should receive a careful neurological exam including all cranial nerves. A lumbar puncture with CSF examination should be performed in patients with syphilis and ocular complaints.

Compliance with Ethical Requirements Drs. Jessica Cao, Careen Lowder, and Steven Gordon declare that they have no conflict of interest.

References

1. GBD 2015 Mortality and Causes of Death Collaborators. Global, regional, and national life expectancy, all-cause mortality, and cause-specific mortality for 249 causes of death, 1980-2015: a systematic analysis for the Global Burden of Disease Study 2015. Lancet Lond Engl. 2016;388(10053):1459–544.
2. Centers for Disease Control and Prevention. Sexually transmitted disease surveillance 2017: Syphilis [Internet]. https://www.cdc.gov/std/stats17/syphilis.htm
3. Oliver SE, Aubin M, Atwell L, Matthias J, Cope A, Mobley V, et al. Ocular syphilis—eight jurisdictions, United States, 2014–2015. MMWR Morb Mortal Wkly Rep. 2016;65(43):1185–8.
4. Giacani L, Lukehart SA. The endemic treponematoses. Clin Microbiol Rev. 2014;27(1):89–115.
5. Tramont E. Treponema pallidum (Syphilis). In: Mandell G, Bennett J, Dolin R, editors. Principles and practice of infectious diseases. 5th ed. Philadelphia: Churchill Livingstone; 2000. p. 2474–90.
6. Tsuboi M, Nishijima T, Yashiro S, Teruya K, Kikuchi Y, Katai N, et al. Time to development of ocular syphilis after syphilis infection. J Infect Chemother. 2018;24(1):75–7.
7. González-Duarte A, López ZM. Neurological findings in early syphilis: a comparison between HIV positive and negative patients. Neurol Int. 2013;5(4):e19.
8. Rompalo AM, Joesoef MR, O'Donnell JA, Augenbraun M, Brady W, Radolf JD, et al. Clinical manifestations of early syphilis by HIV status and gender: results of the syphilis and HIV study. Sex Transm Dis. 2001;28(3):158–65.
9. Yang P, Zhang N, Li F, Chen Y, Kijlstra A. Ocular manifestations of syphilitic uveitis in Chinese patients. Retina Phila Pa. 2012;32(9):1906–14.
10. De Santis M, De Luca C, Mappa I, Spagnuolo T, Licameli A, Straface G, et al. Syphilis infection during pregnancy: fetal risks and clinical management. Infect Dis Obstet Gynecol. 2012;2012:430585.
11. Khan MS, Kuruppu DK, Popli TA, Moorthy RS, Mackay DD. Unilateral optic neuritis and central retinal vasculitis due to ocular syphilis. Retin Cases Brief Rep Winter. 2020;14(1):35–8.
12. Pless ML, Kroshinsky D, LaRocque RC, Buchbinder BR, Duncan LM. Case records of the Massachusetts General Hospital. Case 26-2010. A 54-year-old man with loss of vision and a rash. N Engl J Med. 2010;363(9):865–74.
13. Eccleston K, Collins L, Higgins SP. Primary syphilis. Int J STD AIDS. 2008;19(3):145–51.
14. Sparling P, Swartz M, Musher D, Healy B. Sexually transmitted diseases. 4th ed. New York City: McGraw Medical; 2008. p. 661–84.
15. Mullooly C, Higgins SP. Secondary syphilis: the classical triad of skin rash, mucosal ulceration and lymphadenopathy. Int J STD AIDS. 2010;21(8):537–45.
16. STD Surveillance Case Definitions Effective [Internet]. Centers for Disease Control and Prevention; 2014. http://www.cdc.gov/std/stats/CaseDefinitions-2014.pdf
17. de Voux A, Kidd S, Torrone EA. Reported cases of neurosyphilis among early syphilis cases—United States, 2009 to 2015. Sex Transm Dis. 2018;45(1):39–41.
18. Ropper AH. Neurosyphilis. Longo DL, editor. N Engl J Med. 2019;381(14):1358–63.
19. Tamesis RR, Foster CS. Ocular syphilis. Ophthalmology. 1990;97(10):1281–7.
20. Chao JR, Khurana RN, Fawzi AA, Reddy HS, Rao NA. Syphilis: reemergence of an old adversary. Ophthalmology. 2006;113(11):2074–9.
21. Moradi A, Salek S, Daniel E, Gangaputra S, Ostheimer TA, Burkholder BM, et al. Clinical features and incidence rates of ocular complications in patients with ocular syphilis. Am J Ophthalmol. 2015;159(2):334–43.e1
22. Mathew RG, Goh BT, Westcott MC. British Ocular Syphilis Study (BOSS): 2-year national surveillance study of intraocular inflammation secondary to ocular syphilis. Invest Ophthalmol Vis Sci. 2014;55(8):5394–400.
23. Amaratunge BC, Camuglia JE, Hall AJ. Syphilitic uveitis: a review of clinical manifestations and treatment outcomes of syphilitic uveitis in human immunodeficiency virus-positive and negative patients. Clin Exp Ophthalmol. 2010;38(1):68–74.
24. Tsui E, Gal-Or O, Ghadiali Q, Freund KB. Multimodal imaging adds new insights into acute syphilitic pos-

terior placoid chorioretinitis. Retin Cases Brief Rep. 2018;12(Suppl 1):S3–8.
25. Schlaen A, Aquino MP, Ormaechea MS, Couto C, Saravia M. Spectral optical coherence tomography findings in an adult patient with syphilitic bilateral posterior uveitis and unilateral punctate inner retinitis. Am J Ophthalmol Case Rep. 2019;15:100489.
26. Workowski KA, Bolan GA, Centers for Disease Control and Prevention. Sexually transmitted diseases treatment guidelines, 2015. MMWR Recomm Rep Morb Mortal Wkly Rep Recomm Rep. 2015;64(RR-03):1–137.
27. Shann S. Treatment of neurosyphilis with ceftriaxone. Sex Transm Infect. 2003;79(5):415–6.

4 Fungal Infections

Jordan D. Deaner, Eric Cober, and Sumit Sharma

Abbreviations

AIDS	acquired immunodeficiency syndrome
CNS	central nervous system
HIV	human immunodeficiency virus
LASIK	laser-assisted in situ keratomileusis
OCT	optical coherence tomography

Introduction

The distinct anatomic structure of the human eye with both direct exposure to the outside world and a dense capillary network within the choroid plexus places it at distinct risk for infection from both external penetrating trauma and internal disseminated disease. Fungi are a unique group of microorganisms that can take advantage of this ophthalmic anatomy through contaminated penetrating trauma, direct invasion from infected adjacent ocular structures, or fungemia from a remote colonized source. The ophthalmologist must be able to rapidly identify and appropriately treat intraocular fungal disease, as misdiagnosis or delayed treatment can lead to devastating damage to the eye.

J. D. Deaner
Wills Eye Hospital, Mid Atlantic Retina, Philadelphia, PA, USA
e-mail: jdeaner@midatlanticretina.com

E. Cober
Cleveland Clinic Infectious Diseases, Cleveland, OH, USA
e-mail: cobere@ccf.org

S. Sharma (✉)
Cleveland Clinic Cole Eye Institute, Cleveland, OH, USA

Endogenous Fungal Chorioretinitis and Endophthalmitis

Route of Entry

The majority of fungal endophthalmitis occurs secondary to hematogenous dissemination in patients with fungemia and identifiable risk factors. *Candida* and *Aspergillus* species are the two most common causes of endogenous endophthalmitis [1]; however, a variety of other fungi have been reported to cause endophthalmitis as well. The risk of developing endogenous fungal endophthalmitis after fungemia is highly variable throughout the literature, but has been reported to be as high as 37% in patients with untreated candidemia [2]. Subsequent to hematogenous access, the fungus seeds at the level of the choroid and then invades through the retina into the vitreous [3, 4]. Although this is the typical pattern of fungal spread, there are phenotypic nuances by fungal species, with *Candida* having a predisposition to vitreous invasion and *Aspergillus* preferring to

© Springer Nature Switzerland AG 2023
C. Y. Lowder et al. (eds.), *Emerging Ocular Infections*, Essentials in Ophthalmology,
https://doi.org/10.1007/978-3-031-24559-6_4

occupy the chorioretinal interface [3]. Risk factors for fungemia and consequent endogenous fungal endophthalmitis include parenteral nutrition, indwelling intravenous catheter, organ transplantation, immunomodulatory therapy, neutropenia, diabetes, long-term systemic antibiotic use, abdominal surgery, recent abortion, intravenous drug abuse, and endocarditis [3, 5–7].

Clinical Features

Patients with endogenous fungal infections have a wide range of presenting symptoms, from asymptomatic infection to critical illness, and are often unable to verbally or physically express ophthalmic symptoms. The most common symptoms of endogenous fungal ocular infection include blurred vision, floaters, photophobia, and a red, painful eye [3, 5–7].

In one large study of 370 patients with systemic fungemia, 40 patients were diagnosed with probable ocular infection with 34 (84%) of these patients having chorioretinitis and only 6 (16%) patients developing endophthalmitis [8]. On dilated fundus examination, early endogenous infections typically show small creamy-white lesions at the level of the choroid and retina [4]. Chorioretinitis lesions secondary to *Candida* infection are more likely to be small, multifocal, and distributed throughout the retina (Fig. 4.1a) [3]. *Aspergillus* lesions tend to be confluent, larger, and associated with vascular occlusion and retinal hemorrhages due to its angioinvasive predilection (Fig. 4.2) [3]. These retinal hemorrhages may surround the focal areas of chorioretinitis and should not be confused with Roth spots. As the chorioretinal lesions expand and invade the vitreous cavity, they develop hazy borders (Fig. 4.3) [6]. These chorioretinal lesions may become progressively more difficult to see as the disease progresses due to increasing vitreous involvement and haze (Fig. 4.4). Classically, as the fungus invades the vitreous, it creates vitreous abscesses and gives a characteristic "string of pearls" appearance that can help narrow the differential diagnosis (Fig. 4.5). Fungal endophthalmitis can be associated with varying levels of anterior chamber cell, flare, and a hypopyon [6]. The overall ocular course of fungal endophthalmitis tends to be more indolent, progressing slowly compared to bacterial endophthalmitis. Patients may lack systemic symptoms at time of endophthalmitis diagnosis, particularly when the mode of acquisition is underlying injection drug use. In such cases, transient fungemia can lead to endophthalmitis with a complete absence of systemic symptoms. Hospitalized patients with critical illness or endocarditis often will be febrile and display signs of sepsis.

The differential diagnosis of endogenous fungal endophthalmitis includes, but is not limited to, non-infectious multifocal choroiditis and panuveitis, herpetic and cytomegaloviral retinitis, bacterial endophthalmitis, toxoplasma chorioretinitis, syphilis, and primary vitreoretinal lymphoma.

Diagnostic Work-Up

Cultures should be obtained directly from the vitreous cavity or anterior chamber when they are visibly involved [9, 10]. Fungal cultures should also be obtained from suspected sources, including peripheral blood cultures and samples from central venous and other indwelling catheters. Blood cultures are often negative at the time of diagnosis but should be obtained because the presence of fungemia would have implications for treatment, particularly if concurrent endocarditis is present. Suspected fungal endophthalmitis without a clear exogenous source should be considered a marker for disseminated infection and requires further systemic evaluation and work-up guided by symptoms. In patients with *Candida* endophthalmitis, a transthoracic echocardiogram (TTE) should be obtained to assess for endocarditis. A transesophageal echocardiogram (TEE) can be considered if there are abnormalities on the TTE or the TTE is of poor quality due to body habitus, but is not required in all patients. Vitrectomy can be useful both diagnostically, by allowing for further cultures and pathologic examination, and therapeutically by decreasing the total infectious burden [3, 11]. Although not routinely performed, a retinal

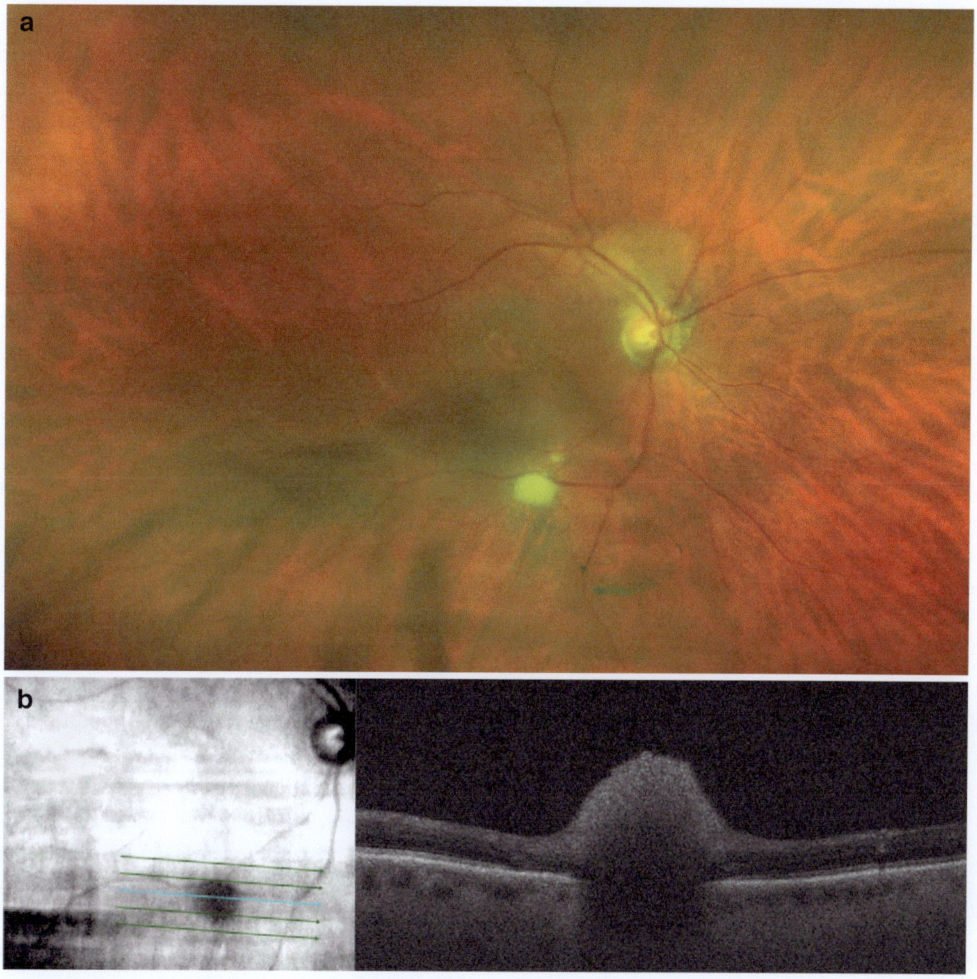

Fig. 4.1 Fundus photograph demonstrating two small chorioretinal lesions along the inferior arcade with associated vitritis in a patient with systemic *Candida* fungemia (**a**). Near infrared and optical coherence tomography through the larger lesion reveals a full thickness involvement of the retina and underlying choroid (**b**)

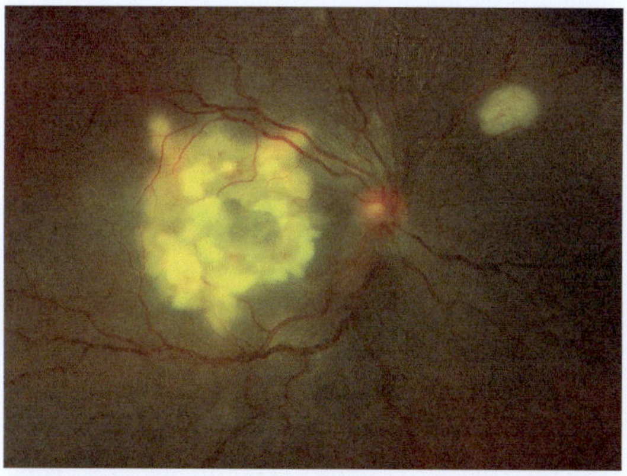

Fig. 4.2 Fundus photograph of a young boy with systemic aspergillosis revealing a large subretinal lesion and a smaller focus superonasal to the optic nerve

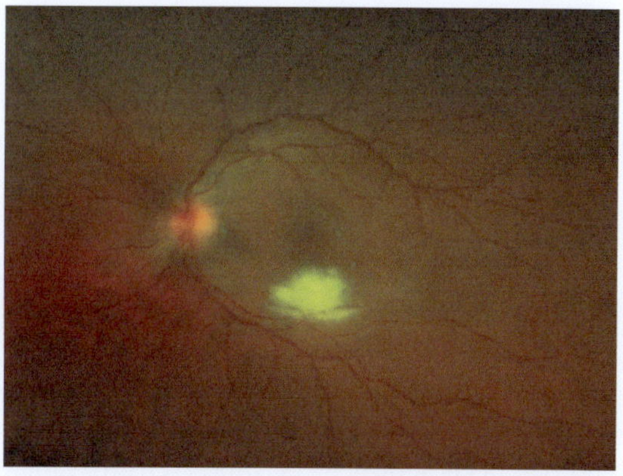

Fig. 4.3 Fundus photograph revealing a large chorioretinal fungal lesion in the inferior macula with multiple smaller satellite lesions that are beginning to invade the vitreous

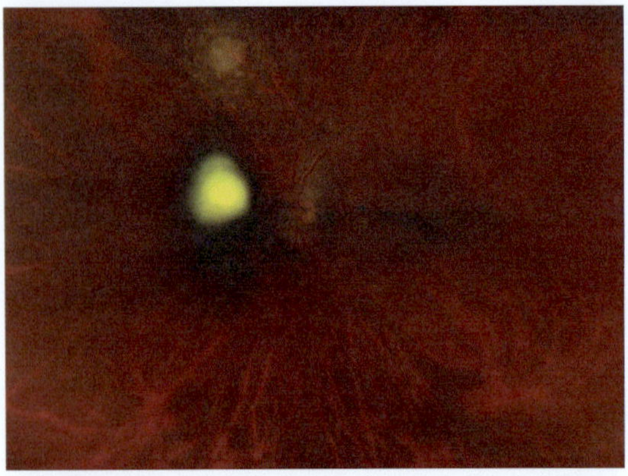

Fig. 4.4 Fundus photograph showing a large vitreous fungal ball emanating from a chorioretinal lesion superior to the optic nerve in a patient with systemic *Candida* fungemia

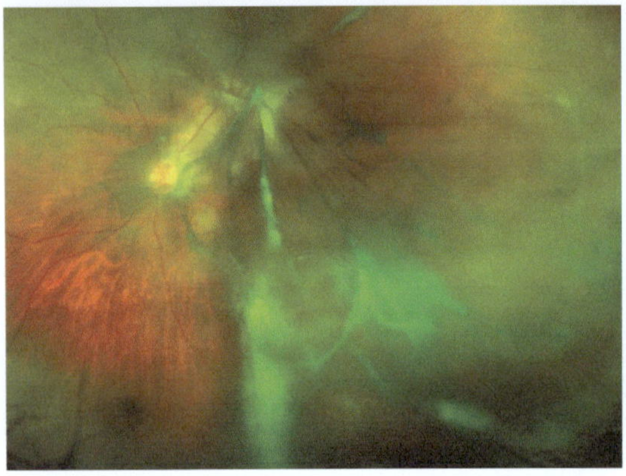

Fig. 4.5 Fundus photograph demonstrating dense vitreous strands, often referred to as a "string of pearls", emanating from a large chorioretinal lesion adjacent to the optic nerve in a patient with systemic *Candid*a fungemia

biopsy can be obtained for culture and histopathologic examination in atypical cases or cases not responsive to antifungal therapy. Microscopic examination of the biopsied or cultured material can be stained with Gomori methenamine silver (GMS), Calcofluor white, or periodic acid-Schiff (PAS) to help identify the causative branching fungi or budding yeast [3]. Although not widely available, polymerase chain reaction can be performed on vitreous or anterior chamber samples and has been shown to be more sensitive than cultures [12]. Optical coherence tomography (OCT) may be useful in discriminating between species of fungal infection. OCT imaging of *Candida* lesions typically demonstrates variable presentations including subretinal, inner retinal, sub-inner limiting membrane, and full thickness lesions (Fig. 4.1b), while *Aspergillus* lesions preferentially demonstrate subretinal lesions with a relatively intact overlying retina [13, 14]. OCT and fluorescein angiography may be used to follow disease activity or assess for possible sequelae such as choroidal neovascularization.

Management

Treatment of fungal endophthalmitis includes systemic antifungal agents for all patients guided by blood and ocular cultures and depending on the site of infection within the eye local intraocular control with intravitreal or intracameral antifungal agents [11]. Consultation with Infectious Disease is advised for selecting systemic antifungal therapy based on the specific organism cultured.

For *Candida* endophthalmitis, fluconazole administered orally is the agent of choice for susceptible *Candida* isolates (including most *C. albicans*, *C. parapsilosis*, *C. tropicalis*, and some *C. glabrata* isolates if demonstrated susceptibility on testing). Fluconazole is given as a loading dose of 800 mg by mouth followed by 400–800 mg daily by mouth. For non-fluconazole-susceptible *Candida* species (i.e., *Candida krusei* and many isolates of *Candida glabrata)*, voriconazole is the preferred agent if susceptibility of the isolate is demonstrated. Voriconazole is given as a loading dose of 6 mg/kg (usually 400 mg) twice daily for two doses followed by 4 mg/kg (usually 200 mg) twice daily. Either the oral or intravenous formulations of voriconazole may be appropriate depending on the acuteness of presentation and whether the patient is being treated in an ambulatory or hospital setting. There is marked inter-patient variability in voriconazole metabolism, and subsequent dosing should be guided by trough levels obtained 5–7 days following initiation of therapy. Patients should be counseled that voriconazole is frequently accompanied by visual disturbances and/or hallucinations, although these often diminish with subsequent doses and in most circumstances are not a reason to discontinue therapy. For non-fluconazole- and non-voriconazole-susceptible *Candida* isolates, liposomal amphotericin B is recommended and is given as an intravenous infusion of 3–5 mg/kg daily. Liposomal amphotericin B is commonly associated with infusion reactions, pronounced renal toxicity, and severe electrolyte disturbances. Initial therapy should be undertaken with close monitoring and in consultation with physicians familiar with its use. Pre-infusion hydration with normal saline and close monitoring of renal function, potassium, and magnesium are recommended. Echinocandins (micafungin, caspofungin, anidulafungin) are generally well tolerated and have a better side effect profile than liposomal amphotericin B but have poor penetration into the vitreous. They have been used in some circumstances in which an isolated chorioretinitis without significant vitreous involvement is present and should only be used with caution and close clinical monitoring for therapeutic response.

For endogenous mold endophthalmitis, systemic voriconazole is recommended for those mold species with expected susceptibility, such as *Aspergillus* and *Fusarium* species. Susceptibility testing for molds can be performed but is generally less available and with slower reporting of results compared to *Candida*. Voriconazole dosing and monitoring considerations are the same as for treatment of *Candida* endophthalmitis. For endogenous endophthalmitis with molds likely resistant to voriconazole, intravenous liposomal amphotericin B is an alternative but with a much greater potential for toxicity. Intravitreal or intracameral amphotericin B (10 μg/0.1 mL) and voriconazole (100 μg/0.1 mL) are the preferred antifungals [15]. Concomitant intravitreal injection of dexamethasone can be performed at the time of antifungal injection with reported retrospective success [16], but is controversial due to limited scientific evidence. If intravitreal steroids are used, dexamethasone is favored due to its short half-life making it unlikely to outlast the duration of the intravitreal antifungals. Severe cases with significant vitreous involvement or progression despite adequate therapy should be taken to the operating room for a combined therapeutic and diagnostic pars plana vitrectomy [3, 11]. Of note, isolated chorioretinal lesions without vitreous involvement can be treated with oral azole antifungals alone and serial examination [15]. The ocular prognosis is variable and dependent on prompt delivery of antifungal therapy, location of chorioretinal involvement, and associated comorbid conditions.

Exogenous Fungal Endophthalmitis

Route of Entry

Exogenous fungal endophthalmitis is less common than its endogenous counterpart. It has been proposed that exogenous fungal infection prevalence varies by climate with warmer, more tropical locations having a higher rate of culture-positive infection [17]. In exogenous infections, the fungus is seeded into the eye by a preceding fungal keratitis, penetrating trauma, or intraocular surgery [6, 18]. Overall, filamentous fungi are the most frequently identified causative microorganism in comparison to yeast [18]. *Fusarium* species are the most commonly isolated organism in endophthalmitis caused by contiguous spread from an infected corneal ulcer [18]. The etiology of the primary fungal keratitis is broad, but risk factors include soft contact lens wear, laser-assisted in situ keratomileusis (LASIK) surgery, penetrating keratoplasty, and non-penetrating trauma from organic debris [6, 18]. Postoperative fungal endophthalmitis occurs most commonly after cataract extraction with intraocular lens implantation but may occur after any intraocular surgery [18]. *Aspergillus* is the most commonly identified species in postoperative cases [18]. Species isolated from previously ruptured globes include *Candida*, *Aspergillus*, and other more exotic species [18]. In comparison to bacterial endophthalmitis, exogenous fungal endophthalmitis often has a latency period prior to the diagnosis which can range from days to months after the inciting event [18].

Clinical Features

Patients with exogenous fungal endophthalmitis present with similar symptoms to their endogenous counterpart including blurred vision, floaters, photophobia, and a red, painful eye. They are uncommonly immunocompromised [18]. A careful history and physical exam must be performed checking for subtle trauma. Careful attention should be paid to the penetrating or surgical site. The infiltrate associated with fungal keratitis classically has a feathered margin and can be associated with immunoglobulin deposition around the borders of the ulcer (Wessely ring) [6]. Associated findings include variable levels of anterior chamber inflammation that may manifest as a hypopyon. The overall course of fungal exogenous endophthalmitis tends to be more indolent and progresses slowly when compared to its bacterial counterpart.

The differential diagnosis overlaps somewhat with that of endogenous endophthalmitis, but additionally includes exogenous bacterial endophthalmitis, lens-induced uveitis, severe postoperative inflammation, sympathetic ophthalmia, and uveitis-glaucoma-hyphema (UGH) syndrome.

Diagnostic Work-Up

Diagnostic evaluation is similar to endogenous fungal endophthalmitis with close attention paid to the etiologic source. Cultures should be obtained directly from the vitreous cavity or anterior chamber when they are involved [9, 10]. If present, infected surgical wounds and corneal ulcers should be cultured on blood agar or Sabouraud dextrose agar [6, 11]. Infected tissue may be biopsied for microscopic examination in culture-negative cases [6, 11]. As in endogenous cases, vitrectomy can be useful both therapeutically and diagnostically.

Management

Treatment of exogenous fungal endophthalmitis includes local intraocular control with intravitreal or intracameral antifungal agents [11]. Amphotericin B (10 μg/0.1 mL) and voriconazole (100 μg/0.1 mL) are the preferred intravitreal antifungals [11]. Systemic antifungals with high intravitreal penetration, i.e., fluconazole or voriconazole depending on the particular fungal species, should be administered with the administration and monitoring considerations already discussed above for endogenous endophthalmitis [18]. Severe cases with significant vitreous involvement or progression despite adequate therapy should be taken to the operating room for a combined therapeutic and diagnostic pars plana vitrectomy [3, 11]. Exogenous infections require additional treatment dependent on the etiology. Fungal keratitis is most commonly caused by filamentous fungal species (particularly *Fusarium*) and responds well to topical natamycin 5% drops [19]. Topical amphotericin B 0.15% drops are efficacious in treating *Candida* keratitis [19]. Topical fortified voriconazole 1% has good coverage of both yeast and filamentous fungi [19]. Perforating injuries need to be primarily repaired or grafted if necessary. Prognosis is variable and dependent on expedited diagnosis, prompt delivery of antifungal therapy, location of ocular involvement, and associated comorbid conditions. Of note, there is a particularly poor prognosis associated with exogenous fungal endophthalmitis after ruptured globe, with up to 70% of cases eventually ending in enucleation [18].

Cryptococcosis

Route of Entry

Cryptococcus neoformans is an encapsulated yeast that is found ubiquitously in soil and avian feces [20]. Primary inoculation occurs when the microorganism is inhaled into the respiratory system where it can cause asymptomatic pulmonary lesions [20]. Subsequent granulomas sequester dormant yeast which can reactivate if the patient becomes immunosuppressed and loses cell-mediated immune response [20]. *Cryptococcus* most likely reaches the eye by hematogenous spread from the lungs where it then seeds at the level of the choriocapillaris [21]. However, direct optic nerve invasion in patients with meningoencephalitis is a theorized route of invasion and may be the reason for rapid loss of vision in certain patients [22]. Disseminated cryptococcal infections occur almost exclusively in immunosuppressed patients, particularly those with HIV or AIDS, prolonged courses of high-dose corticosteroids, and organ and bone marrow transplant recipients [20, 23]. Symptomatic infection in immunocompetent hosts remains uncommon and when present is often limited to the lungs without systemic dissemination [23].

Clinical Features

Patients may present with varying severity of disease, from completely asymptomatic to comorbid disabling central nervous system (CNS) disease [23]. Patients with ocular disease most commonly complain of blurred vision, sudden vision loss, floaters, and photophobia [24]. The most common ocular manifestation of cryptococcosis is optic nerve edema secondary to increased intracranial pressure from meningoencephalitis. [24] Occasionally primary intraocular infection can precede CNS involvement [24]. The most common manifestation of primary intraocular infection is a multifocal choroiditis which can be bilateral in up to 50% of cases (Fig. 4.6) [24]. Associated findings include optic nerve edema, retinitis, vitritis, vasculitis, and exudative retinal detachment [24]. Severe infection can progress to endophthalmitis with an accompanying granulomatous anterior uveitis [24]. Patients with intraocular cryptococcal infections have concomitant meningoencephalitis in up to 81% of cases [24].

The differential for cryptococcosis includes atypical mycobacterial infection, endogenous fungal or bacterial endophthalmitis, vitreoretinal lymphoma, non-infectious multifocal choroiditis and panuveitis, sarcoidosis, syphilis, toxoplasmosis, and tuberculosis.

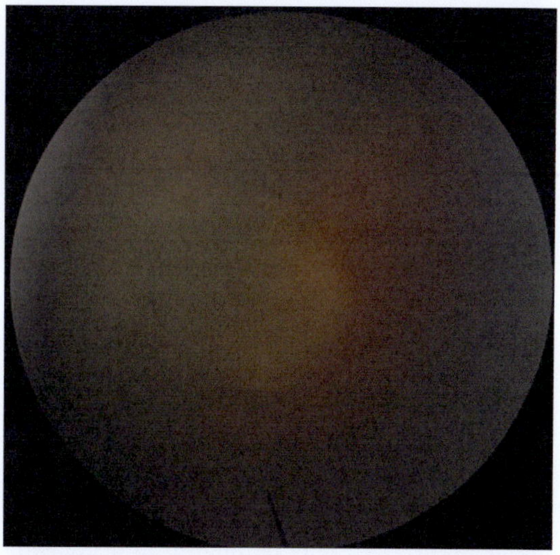

Fig. 4.6 Fundus photograph revealing a superonasal chorioretinal cryptococcoma with overlying vitreous haze in an HIV negative patient with disseminated *Cryptococcus* infection (Reprinted with permission from Springer; Kresch ZA, Espinosa-Heidmann D, Harper T, Miller JG. Disseminated *Cryptococcus* with ocular cryptococcoma in a human immunodeficiency virus-negative patient. *Int Ophthalmol*. 2012;32:281–284)

Diagnostic Work-Up

Cultures and microscopic evaluation of aqueous or vitreous samples should be performed when they are involved, and the diagnosis is in question [24]. If necessary, diagnostic vitrectomy with or without lesion biopsy may be useful in unusual or unresponsive cases though it is an invasive procedure [24]. GMS, PAS, Alcian blue, and mucicarmine stains can be used to identify the yeast on microscopy [23]. OCT imaging of a chorioretinal lesion shows choroidal thickening and hyperreflective lesions at the level of the photoreceptors [25]. Intravenous fluorescein angiography can demonstrate early hypofluorescent spots that stain late, corresponding to the granulomatous inflammation seen on clinical exam [25]. More commonly *Cryptococcus* is identified on systemic work-up [24]. If ocular cryptococcosis is identified first, then the ensuing systemic work-up should include serum cryptococcal antigen, fungal blood cultures, computed tomography of chest, and lumbar puncture with CSF analysis, cryptococcal antigen, opening, pressure, and fungal cultures.

Management

Systemic treatment of cryptococcosis should be undertaken in consultation with infectious disease experts and is beyond the scope of this text. Intravitreal amphotericin B (10 μg/0.1 mL) or voriconazole (100 μg/0.1 mL) can be used as adjuvant therapy to systemic antifungals with severe or macula threatening disease [24]. Vitrectomy, although uncommonly reported in the literature [24], may be helpful in decreasing the infectious burden.

Coccidioidomycosis

Route of Entry

Coccidioides is a dimorphic fungus that is endemic to the southwestern United States, northern Mexico, and South America [26]. Inhaled aerosolized spores result in pulmonary coccidioidomycosis, and from the lungs the fungus can hematogenously disseminate to other parts of the body, including the eye [26]. Increased risk populations for disseminated disease include those of Filipino, Native American, Mexican, and African ancestry, pregnant women, and immunocompromised individuals [27].

Clinical Features

Ocular coccidioidomycosis can equally present as an isolated anterior uveitis [28], posterior uveitis, or more rarely an endophthalmitis [29]. The anterior uveitis may be unilateral or bilateral and is classically granulomatous with prominent "mutton-fat" keratic precipitates [27]. It may be associated with iris granulomas [27, 28, 30]. The posterior segment manifestations are more protean and may entail a diffuse choroiditis, peripapillary chorioretinitis, or multifocal chorioretinitis [27]. Associated findings include variable vitritis, vascular sheathing, and exudative retinal detachment [27]. Disseminated disease can also affect other ocular structures causing conjunctivitis, keratitis, scleritis, blepharitis, extraocular nerve palsies, and orbital infection [27].

Coccidioidomycosis often presents as a subclinical or unrecognized community-acquired pneumonia syndrome. More severe and diffuse pulmonary involvement can occur in a subset of patients. Often, systemic symptoms such as profound fatigue, fevers, night sweats, arthralgias, and cutaneous manifestations can be more pronounced and prolonged than the pulmonary symptoms and do not necessarily imply disseminated disease. Coccidioides can disseminate and cause meningitis, spondylodiskitis, septic arthritis, and skin lesions.

In additional to endogenous fungal endophthalmitis, the differential diagnosis includes other non-infectious and infectious causes of granulomatous uveitis such as sarcoidosis and tuberculosis, respectively, syphilis, and masquerade syndromes such as vitreoretinal lymphoma.

Diagnostic Work-Up

Fluorescein angiography may demonstrate late staining of active choroidal granulomas [31]. OCT angiography has been shown to reveal signal voids in the areas of choroidal lesions [32]. Diagnosis is based upon culture, microscopic, or immunologic demonstration of the causative fungus, either locally or systemically [31]. The microscopic finding of fungal spherules with endospores is pathognomonic for *Coccidioides* infection [33]. Samples of aqueous and vitreous may be sent for culture and microscopic evaluation if they are involved. The detection of *Coccidioides* by real-time PCR has also been explored [34]. Diagnostic vitrectomy with or without chorioretinal granuloma biopsy may be useful in unusual or unresponsive cases to secure a diagnosis. Diagnosis can be additionally supported by serological and antigen testing. An enzyme-linked immunoassay is available for screening and, if positive, should be followed by immunodiffusion testing. Urine and blood antigens are also available for the detection of *Coccidioides*.

Management

Systemic antifungal therapy is the standard of care for ocular coccidioidomycosis as it is indicative of disseminated disease. Initial therapy consists of fluconazole given as a loading dose of 800 mg by mouth followed by 400–800 mg daily by mouth. Intravitreal amphotericin B (10 μg/0.1 mL) may be used as adjuvant therapy, especially in cases of endophthalmitis. However, this is not well established in the literature [28]. Vitrectomy may be done in recalcitrant or severe cases. Prognosis is dependent on the severity of ocular involvement. Anterior disease can cause subsequent cataract, posterior synechiae, and secondary angle closure glaucoma [31]. Posterior disease can cause an exudative retinal detachment, resultant epiretinal membrane, and choroidal neovascular membranes [31]. Disease directly involving the macula or optic nerve can be visually devastating [31].

Pneumocystosis

Route of Entry

Pneumocystis jirovecii (previously known as *Pneumocystis carinii*) primarily affects the lungs of immunocompromised patients (receipt of systemic corticosteroids, solid organ and bone marrow transplant recipients, and HIV patients with CD4 counts below 200/μL) [35–37]. Subsequent systemic dissemination from the lungs leads to infection of other parts of the body, including the eyes [35–37]. Ocular involvement was predominantly diagnosed in patients who were on aerosolized pentamidine prophylaxis against *Pneumocystis jirovecii* [35–37]. Aerosolized pentamidine has since been recognized as a risk factor for dissemination, and its use is no longer recommended [35–37].

Clinical Features

Dilated fundus examination in *Pneumocystis* choroiditis demonstrates multifocal deep yellow lesions at the level of the choroid with minimal or absent associated vitritis [35–37]. These lesions are typically limited to the posterior pole [35–37]. Both eyes may be involved in up to 76% of cases [37]. As *Pneumocystis* typically causes an isolated choroiditis with minimal inflammation, most patients are asymptomatic unless the macula is involved [35].

The differential diagnosis of *Pneumocystis jirovecii*-associated endophthalmitis includes the aforementioned endogenous endophthalmitides, uveitides known to cause subretinal and choroidal lesions such as sarcoidosis and tuberculosis, and masquerade syndromes such as lymphoma and metastasis.

Diagnostic Work-Up

Fluorescein angiography typically shows early hypofluorescence of the choroidal lesions, followed by late staining [37]. Diagnosis is typically made on clinical examination in the context of high clinical suspicion in a patient with known or suspected clinical risk factors.

Management

A diagnosis of *Pneumocystis* choroiditis is suggestive of disseminated disease and requires systemic treatment. The ocular prognosis is typically good if there is good response to systemic therapy.

The preferred treatment regimen is intravenous trimethoprim-sulfamethoxazole (20 mg/kg/day of trimethoprim component) divided into three to four doses, which can be transitioned to oral trimethoprim-sulfamethoxazole once improvement is noted, for a total duration of 21 days, followed by secondary prophylaxis until resolution of underlying risk factors [35–37]. For patients intolerant of trimethoprim-sulfamethoxazole, treatment should be undertaken in consultation with infectious disease experts and is beyond the scope of this text.

Conflicts of Interest None of the authors has disclosures related to the submitted work.

Dr. Sharma has the following disclosures outside of the submitted work: Consultant for Alimera, Allergan, Bausch & Lomb, Clearside, Eyepoint, Genentech/Roche, and Regeneron; Research Support from Gilead, Genentech/Roche, Santen, and IONIS.

Dr. Deaner has the following disclosures outside the submitted work: 2020–2021 Heed Fellow supported by the Heed Ophthalmic Foundation and Advisory board and received honorarium from Alimera Sciences, Inc.

References

1. Essman TF, Flynn HW, Smiddy WE, Brod RD, Murray TG, Davis JL, et al. Treatment outcomes in a 10-year study of endogenous fungal endophthalmitis. Ophthalmic Surg Lasers. 1997;28(3):185–94.
2. Parke DW, Jones DB, Gentry LO. Endogenous endophthalmitis among patients with candidemia. Ophthalmology. 1982;89(7):789–96.
3. Rao NA, Hidayat AA. Endogenous mycotic endophthalmitis: variations in clinical and histopathologic changes in candidiasis compared with aspergillosis. Am J Ophthalmol. 2001;132(2):244–51.
4. Samiy N, D'Amico DJ. Endogenous fungal endophthalmitis. Int Ophthalmol Clin. 1996;36(3):147–62.
5. Kato H, Yoshimura Y, Suido Y, Ide K, Sugiyama Y, Matsuno K, et al. Prevalence of, and risk factors for, hematogenous fungal endophthalmitis in patients with Candida bloodstream infection. Infection. 2018;46(5):635–40.
6. Klotz SA, Penn CC, Negvesky GJ, Butrus SI. Fungal and parasitic infections of the eye. Clin Microbiol Rev. 2000;13(4):662–85.
7. Shah CP, McKey J, Spirn MJ, Maguire J. Ocular candidiasis: a review. Br J Ophthalmol. 2008;92(4):466–8.
8. Oude Lashof AML, Rothova A, Sobel JD, Ruhnke M, Pappas PG, Viscoli C, et al. Ocular manifestations of candidemia. Clin Infect Dis Off Publ Infect Dis Soc Am. 2011;53(3):262–8.
9. Tamai M, Nakazawa M. A collection system to obtain vitreous humor in clinical cases. Arch Ophthalmol Chic Ill 1960. 1991;109(4):465–6.
10. Koul S, Philipson A, Arvidson S. Role of aqueous and vitreous cultures in diagnosing infectious endophthalmitis in rabbits. Acta Ophthalmol. 1990;68(4):466–9.
11. Vilela RC, Vilela L, Vilela P, Vilela R, Motta R, Pôssa AP, et al. Etiological agents of fungal endophthalmitis: diagnosis and management. Int Ophthalmol. 2014;34(3):707–21.
12. Anand AR, Madhavan HN, Neelam V, Lily TK. Use of polymerase chain reaction in the diagnosis of fungal endophthalmitis. Ophthalmology. 2001;108(2):326–30.
13. Zhuang H, Ding X, Gao F, Zhang T, Ni Y, Chang Q, et al. Optical coherence tomography features of retinal lesions in Chinese patients with endogenous Candida endophthalmitis. BMC Ophthalmol. 2020;20(1):52.
14. Adam CR, Sigler EJ. Multimodal imaging findings in endogenous aspergillus endophthalmitis. Retina Phila Pa. 2014;34(9):1914–5.
15. Riddell J, Comer GM, Kauffman CA. Treatment of endogenous fungal Endophthalmitis: focus on new antifungal agents. Clin Infect Dis. 2011;52(5):648–53.
16. Chakrabarti A, Shivaprakash MR, Singh R, Tarai B, George VK, Fomda BA, et al. Fungal endophthalmitis: fourteen years' experience from a center in India. Retina Phila Pa. 2008;28(10):1400–7.
17. Kunimoto DY, Das T, Sharma S, Jalali S, Majji AB, Gopinathan U, et al. Microbiologic spectrum and susceptibility of isolates: part II. Posttraumatic endophthalmitis. Am J Ophthalmol. 1999;128(2):242–4.
18. Wykoff CC, Flynn HW, Miller D, Scott IU, Alfonso EC. Exogenous fungal Endophthalmitis: microbiology and clinical outcomes. Ophthalmology. 2008;115(9):1501–1507.e2.
19. Sahay P, Singhal D, Nagpal R, Maharana PK, Farid M, Gelman R, et al. Pharmacologic therapy of mycotic keratitis. Surv Ophthalmol. 2019;64(3):380–400.
20. May RC, Stone NRH, Wiesner DL, Bicanic T, Nielsen K. Cryptococcus: from environmental saprophyte to global pathogen. Nat Rev Microbiol. 2016;14(2):106–17.
21. Chapman-Smith JS. Cryptococcal chorioretinitis: a case report. Br J Ophthalmol. 1977;61(6):411–3.
22. Merkler AE, Gaines N, Baradaran H, Schuetz AN, Lavi E, Simpson SA, et al. Direct invasion of the optic nerves, chiasm, and tracts by Cryptococcus neoformans in an immunocompetent host. Neurohospitalist. 2015;5(4):217–22.
23. Góralska K, Blaszkowska J, Dzikowiec M. Neuroinfections caused by fungi. Infection. 2018;46(4):443–59.
24. Crump JRC, Elner SG, Elner VM, Kauffman CA. Cryptococcal Endophthalmitis: case report and review. Clin Infect Dis. 1992;14(5):1069–73.
25. Aderman CM, Gorovoy IR, Chao DL, Bloomer MM, Obeid A, Stewart JM. Cryptococcal choroiditis in advanced AIDS with clinicopathologic correlation. Am J Ophthalmol Case Rep. 2018;10:51–4.
26. Ampel NM. Coccidioidomycosis: changing concepts and knowledge gaps. J Fungi [Internet]. 2020;6(4) [cited 2021 Jan 25]; Available from: https://www.ncbi.nlm.nih.gov/pmc/articles/PMC7770576/
27. Rodenbiker HT, Ganley JP. Ocular coccidioidomycosis. Surv Ophthalmol. 1980;24(5):263–90.
28. Moorthy RS, Rao NA, Sidikaro Y, Foos RY. Coccidioidomycosis Iridocyclitis. Ophthalmology. 1994 Dec;101(12):1923–8.

29. Vasconcelos-Santos DV, Lim JI, Rao NA. Chronic Coccidioidomycosis Endophthalmitis without concomitant systemic involvement: a Clinicopathological case report. Ophthalmology. 2010;117(9):1839–42.
30. Bell R, Font RL. Granulomatous anterior uveitis caused by Coccidioides immitis. Am J Ophthalmol. 1972 Jul;74(1):93–8.
31. Jonna G, Agarwal A. Coccidioidomycosis. In: Gupta V, Nguyen QD, LeHoang P, Herbort CP, editors. The uveitis atlas. New Delhi: Springer India; 2018.
32. Shields RA, Tang PH, Bodnar ZM, Smith SJ, Silva AR. Optical coherence tomography angiography highlights Chorioretinal lesions in ocular Coccidioidomycosis. Ophthalmic Surg Lasers Imaging Retina. 2019;50(3):e71–3.
33. Stevens DA. Coccidioidomycosis. N Engl J Med. 1995;332(16):1077–82.
34. Vucicevic D, Blair JE, Binnicker MJ, McCullough AE, Kusne S, Vikram HR, et al. The utility of Coccidioides polymerase chain reaction testing in the clinical setting. Mycopathologia. 2010 Nov;170(5):345–51.
35. Foster RE, Lowder CY, Meisler DM, Huang SS, Longworth DL. Presumed pneumocystis carinii choroiditis: Unifocal presentation, regression with intravenous Pentamidine, and choroiditis recurrence. Ophthalmology. 1991;98(9):1360–5.
36. Sha BE, Benson CA, Deutsch T, Noskin GA, Murphy RL, Pottage JJ, et al. Pneumocystis carinii choroiditis in patients with AIDS: clinical features, response to therapy, and outcome. J Acquir Immune Defic Syndr. 1992;5(10):1051–8.
37. Shami MJ, Freeman W, Friedberg D, Siderides E, Listhaus A, Ai E. A multicenter study of pneumocystis Choroidopathy. Am J Ophthalmol. 1991;112(1):15–22.

Viral Retinitis

5

Carlos Isada, Ryan Miller, Arthi Venkat,
and Rebecca Chen

Introduction

Herpes simplex virus (HSV), varicella zoster virus (VZV), and cytomegalovirus (CMV) are among the most common viral pathogens responsible for infectious retinitis. These viruses can cause chronic anterior uveitis, acute retinal necrosis (ARN), and progressive outer retinal necrosis (PORN), the latter two being responsible in some cases for sequelae such as optic neuropathy, chronic retinal ischemia and retinal detachment. ARN is classically found in immunocompetent patients, whereas PORN is most common in immunocompromised patients, initially coming to light during the human immunodeficiency virus (HIV)-associated acquired immunodeficiency syndrome (AIDS) epidemic.

CMV affects roughly 45% to 100% of the population depending on geography [1]. HSV-1 subtype has been identified in between 45% and 98% of the world population, whereas 40–63% of the United States (US) population has been shown to have antibodies against this virus [2]. Seropositivity increases with age, as expected. It has been shown that lower income and minority groups also have a higher seropositive rate for HSV-1 in the United States [2]. HSV-2 tends to affect fewer people, with 20–25% of the US population having antibodies by 40 years of age [2]. Classically, HSV-1 has been associated with oral HSV lesions and HSV-2 more so with genital lesions; however, this distinction is beginning to blur.

CMV retinitis continues to be problematic especially in hematopoietic stem cell transplant (HSCT) recipients and less so in solid organ transplant (SOT) recipients. Increased levels of immunosuppressive medications pose a clinical challenge for viral reactivation. However, advances in antiviral therapy have offset this risk with preemptive and prophylactic strategies in transplant recipients.

Other viruses that have been implicated to cause ocular infections include chikungunya virus, dengue virus, yellow fever virus (YFV), West Nile virus (WNV), and Zika virus (ZV) [3–5]. WNV is a single-stranded RNA flavivirus which is transmitted by the *Culex* genus of mosquitoes and has been identified in Africa, Europe, Australia, Asia, the United States, Canada, Mexico, Central America, and South America [3]. Patients may develop chorioretinitis, which is associated with concomitant neurologic disease

C. Isada · R. Miller
Department of Infectious Disease, Cleveland Clinic, Cleveland, OH, USA
e-mail: ISADAC@ccf.org; millerr4@ccf.org

A. Venkat (✉)
Department of Ophthalmology - Medical Retina and Uveitis, University of Virginia, Charlottesville, USA
e-mail: arthivenkat@virginia.edu

R. Chen
University of California, Davis, Sacramento, CA, USA

© Springer Nature Switzerland AG 2023
C. Y. Lowder et al. (eds.), *Emerging Ocular Infections*, Essentials in Ophthalmology,
https://doi.org/10.1007/978-3-031-24559-6_5

such as encephalitis. Chikungunya, dengue, and Zika viruses are all arboviruses transmitted by the *Aedes aegypti* mosquito and occasionally other *Aedes* species. Chikungunya virus is an alphavirus, while dengue and Zika viruses belong to the *Flaviviridae* family. These are all single-stranded RNA viruses. Retinitis is less common with these viruses as less than 10% of symptomatic dengue infections have been identified to have ocular manifestations, whereas chikungunya and Zika infections have an even lower prevalence of ocular disease, with only a few cases reported. Treatment of these viruses is limited as there are no active antiviral medications, and symptoms are managed with corticosteroids [3–5].

Pathogenesis

HSV and VZV are neurotropic viruses which cause latent infection by integrating viral genomic material into the host tissue [6]. Chronic latency is then interrupted by periodic reactivation to a variety of internal and external triggers [2]. Patients tend to develop a primary HSV infection of mucocutaneous surfaces from which the virus integrates into the nerve ganglion and remains latent for life. In contrast, VZV primary infection manifests as chickenpox; however, the incidence of this is decreasing significantly due to vaccination campaigns [7]. The predominant theory of the pathogenesis of herpes virus infection is a latent infection in the dorsal root ganglia or trigeminal ganglion with reactivation in specific dermatomes with retrograde movement of the virus [6]. Reactivation has been associated with stressors such as sunlight, trauma, emotional stress, menstruation, or other infections [8]. There has also been suggestion that HSV can remain dormant in corneal nerves after prior keratitis, as it is an immunologically privileged site [9].

Entry of HSV into ocular cells can occur by exogenous exposure to the virus (such as via corneal transplant), local reactivation in the cornea, or reactivated virus that travels anterograde along the ophthalmic division of the trigeminal nerve [9]. Interactions between the nectin-1 receptor and the viral surface glycoprotein gD facilitate endocytosis of HSV-1, 2 into a variety of ocular cell types including retinal pigment epithelial cells and are thought to be the primary mechanism of viral entry [10].

CMV retinitis was described in patients with HIV infection in the early 1980s [11]. It occurred late in the disease course when the CD4+ T-lymphocyte count dropped below 50 cells per microliter. CMV retinitis also occurs in immunocompromised patients such as HSCT recipients [12, 13]. It has also been described in immunocompetent individuals, but this seems to be a much rarer occurrence. The pathogenesis is similar to HSV or VZV, in that it is thought to be reactivation of latent virus that causes the disease. Roughly 56% of Australians between 1 and 59 years of age were found to be seropositive for CMV in a 2006 study [14]. Other than in advanced HIV infection, CMV retinitis has been described in organ transplant recipients. An example of such a case occurred in a deceased donor kidney transplant recipient who had received belatacept [15]. The patient had several episodes of CMV reactivation treated systemically and then developed a multidrug-resistant CMV retinitis with the virus detected in plasma and aqueous humor.

In HSCT recipients, risk of CMV retinitis is determined by recipient CMV IgG status. If the recipient is CMV IgG-positive, denoting the presence of latent CMV infection, there is risk for reactivation. If a CMV IgG-positive recipient receives a HSCT from a CMV IgG-negative donor, the newly acquired immune system will be CMV-naïve putting the recipient at risk for CMV reactivation [16]. The induction and conditioning regimen, which often includes high-dose corticosteroids, T-cell-depleting agents, and treatment for graft-versus-host disease in allogeneic HSCT recipients, may also play a role in patient reactivation [16]. Valganciclovir and letermovir are currently approved for CMV prophylaxis in high-risk groups. Failure of prophylaxis may occur due to inadequate medication adherence, dosing inconsistency, or prophylaxis discontinuation in response to adverse effects of medications (such as pancytopenia). CMV retinitis develops in 11.3% of SOT recipients with CMV viremia [17]. Risk factors for poor prognosis included concurrent systemic CMV disease and foveal involvement in one study. In this study, prevalence of CMV retinitis trended towards lower rates in SOT recipients (8.7%) than HSCT recipients (15.4%), with a p value of 0.052. The mortality rate over the mean 11.7-month follow-up in patients diagnosed with CMV retinitis was 52.4% in HSCT recipients compared to 5.6% in SOT recipients ($p < 0.001$) [17].

In cases of CMV or disseminated herpesvirus infection, the virus enters the eye hematogenously through a compromised blood-retinal barrier [18]. Retinal microvascular endothelial cells are the initial target of CMV infection, and from there CMV spreads to adjacent perivascular glia, Muller cells, and other retinal cells such as the retinal pigment epithelium [18]. The virus infects retinal pigment epithelial cells via their apical membrane and spreads laterally cell-to-cell [19]. In response to viral exposure, infected endothelial cells undergo apoptosis and stimulate the release of pro-inflammatory mediators by neurosensory and glial cells [18]. Tumor necrosis factor-alpha and **interferon-gamma** sensitize the retinal pigment epithelial cells and other retinal cells to undergo FasL-mediated apoptosis [20]. EBV has also been implicated in viral retinitis, though there are only a handful of reported cases with molecular confirmation.

In immunocompetent individuals, the presence of virus in the eye provokes a strong immunologic response from the host, causing infiltration of the vitreous and retina by mononuclear cells. A high proportion of T lymphocytes, particularly CD4+ T cells (70%), were isolated from vitreous sample with acute retinal necrosis [21]. Retinal arteriolar vasculitis results in vascular occlusion and necrosis of downstream retinal tissue.

In contrast to the above infections, the majority of arbovirus-mediated retinitis occurs during the acute infectious phase. Dengue virus has four separate serotypes and typically causes a self-limited flu-like syndrome. However it can manifest as the feared dengue hemorrhagic fever with severe bleeding, respiratory distress, and multiorgan failure, which is more common with repeated infection with a different serotype [3]. Retinitis most commonly manifests within 5–7 days of the initial infection and is thought to be due to an immune-mediated response to the virus. In young adults, ocular manifestations tend to occur at the nadir of thrombocytopenia, the latter of which may be explained by circulatory compromise or immune complex deposition [3].

West Nile-associated retinitis can be seen as commonly as 80% in patients with concomitant neurologic disease [3, 5]. Neurologic complications occur in less than 1% of WN virus infections, however. The pathogenesis is likely due to direct infection and is characterized as multifocal chorioretinitis. Vascular manifestations can occur with retinal hemorrhages, retinal vascular sheathing, vascular leakage, and possibly occlusive retinal vasculitis [3–5].

Chikungunya virus infections typically manifest as fevers, malaise, arthralgia, rash, vomiting, and myalgias, but meningoencephalitis has also been reported [4]. Ocular manifestations can be unilateral or bilateral, and the pathogenesis is unknown. Ocular infections occur concomitantly with systemic disease, so there may be a component of direct infection or immunologic response to the virus driving the ocular manifestations [4].

Zika virus infection manifests as fever, conjunctivitis, and rash and can result in severe birth defects such as microcephaly if primary infection occurs during pregnancy [3]. Macular atrophy from in utero infections has been reported. Acute maculopathy, multifocal choroiditis, and optic neuritis have also been reported in adults [3]. Zika virus has been demonstrated to directly infect multiple retinal cell types and induce apoptosis in animal models.

Clinical Features

Acute retinal necrosis (ARN) and progressive outer retinal necrosis (PORN) describe two patterns that exist along a spectrum of viral necrotizing retinitis. ARN is characterized by multifocal, well-demarcated, peripheral retinal whitening that rapidly coalesces and spreads in a circumferential pattern [22]. It is frequently accompanied by anterior chamber inflammation, occlusive arteriolitis, and prominent vitritis [22]. Concurrent optic nerve involvement can also be seen and can be visually devastating.

HSV encephalitis and acute retinal necrosis may occur concomitantly [23]. Patients may present with new-onset seizures, fevers, or altered mental status, and these features may prompt further work up for encephalitis or meningitis. Often, oral lesions are not associated with concomitant HSV meningitis, encephalitis, or retinitis. The disease presentation is frequently insidious with no prior warning or prodrome.

In PORN, retinal necrosis begins in the outer retina but quickly progresses to full-thickness involvement. In contrast to ARN, the multifocal retinal whitening tends to begin more posteriorly, and there is a relative absence or reduced degree of inflammation in the rest of the eye due to the profound immunosuppression of the host. A characteristic "cracked mud" appearance has been described in PORN owing to a perivascular pattern of retinal sparing, which can be present until late stages of PORN. Angiographic studies have demonstrated sparing of the perivenous capillary network despite concurrent arteriolar attenuation and retinal staining in eyes with diffuse retinal involvement [24].

After resolution of active retinitis, the eye enters the cicatricial phase. Retinal holes or breaks frequently occur at the junction of normal and atrophic retina. Additionally, proliferative vitreoretinopathy develops as a later consequence of the acute immunologic response. Retinal detachment is common, occurring by a combination of rhegmatogenous and tractional mechanisms.

Notably, VZV infection is associated with more aggressive disease and poorer visual outcomes in patients with acute retinal necrosis [25]. Compared to HSV ARN, a lower proportion of patients with VZV ARN presented with good visual acuity (≥20/60), and a higher portion had poor vision (≤20/200) at 1 year. This difference in visual outcome may be mediated by a higher rate of retinal detachment in eyes with VZV ARN [25].

CMV infections may present with a multitude of organ systems involved including pneumonitis, colitis, enteritis, pancreatitis, gastritis, pancytopenia, myocarditis, meningitis, and nephritis [14]. Primary infection most commonly presents as an acute mononucleosis. Retinitis has not been reported in acute infections. CMV retinitis classically presents as one of three pathologic patterns. The "frosted branch angiitis" pattern is characterized by prominent peri-arteriolar sheathing. In the hemorrhagic pattern, retinal hemorrhages and yellow-white necrotic lesions are found, frequently perivascularly. The granular form involves peripheral retinal granularity with minimal frank hemorrhage or necrosis. Compared to ARN and PORN, there is relatively reduced or absent intraocular inflammation due to the underlying immunocompromised status of the host, and the retinitis is typically slower to progress. Consequently, patients with CMV retinitis may sometimes suffer from delayed diagnosis due to fewer or more subtle symptoms, with up to 33% of CMV retinitis patients reporting no symptoms in one case series [24].

Lab Testing

The differential diagnosis of infectious retinitis includes *Toxoplasma gondii*, CMV, HSV, VZV, *Mycobacterium tuberculosis*, and *Treponema pallidum*. If appropriate risk factors are present, such as travel to a known endemic area or a high-volume season for mosquito bites, PCR and antibody testing can be performed for West Nile, dengue, chikungunya, and Zika viruses. Some of these can only be completed by special laboratories or the Centers for Disease Control and Prevention (CDC). Laboratory analysis should be done with the aim of ruling out these causes when possible and should include HIV screen, treponemal and non-treponemal syphilis screens, latent tuberculosis screening through an interferon-gamma release (QuantiFERON) assay, and *T. gondii* serum IgG screen. Brain imaging and cerebrospinal fluid (CSF) analysis should be considered on a case-by-case basis, as encephalitis or meningitis can also present concomitantly with retinitis [26].

Serum CMV levels appear to have limited utility in diagnosing CMV retinitis as they are not sensitive [13]. The same is true of HSV and VZV serology. Although viral retinitis is a clinical diagnosis, molecular confirmation is helpful to determine the etiologic virus and to differentiate from masqueraders such as toxoplasmosis in immunocompromised individuals. Polymerase chain reaction (PCR) testing is the gold standard to confirm the intraocular presence of HSV, VZV, or CMV. An aqueous humor sample is ideal for PCR testing. PCR of an aqueous sample was able to identify HSV or VZV DNA in 79% to 100% of cases with necrotizing retinitis [27, 28]. Given the high sensitivity of PCR using aqueous samples, vitreous tap is not the preferred diagnostic procedure, especially given an increased risk of vitreous traction that may potentiate retinal tears or detachments in already weakened portions of the retina.

In addition to viral PCR, testing for other causes of retinitis should be obtained. Toxoplasmosis in immunocompromised patients can lead to a similar appearance, and therefore an aqueous sample can also be tested for toxoplasma PCR. However, empiric treatment for viral retinitis should not be delayed while awaiting laboratory testing, given the potential for significant and rapid visual morbidity.

Management

A combination of systemic and local therapy forms the mainstay of treatment. Therapy should be initiated at the time of clinical diagnosis and should not be delayed for molecular confirmation.

HSV and VZV Retinitis

The American Academy of Ophthalmology recommendations for antiviral treatment of ARN include systemic acyclovir, valacyclovir, famciclovir, foscarnet, or ganciclovir [27]. Initially, oral or intravenous antivirals can be used based on the preference or experience of the treating physician. A few studies have shown that oral antiviral agents can be effective in reducing progression to retinal detachment [29, 30]. One systematic review focused on retinal detachment after ARN and the efficacies of the published interventions. The conclusion from this study was VZV-associated ARN may require more intensive interventions as the incidence of retinal detachment was higher compared to HSV-associated ARN. Additionally, systemic antivirals are effective and prophylactic vitrectomy may provide benefit [31]. Zhao et al. reviewed retinal detachment in patients with viral retinitis for alternative or additional treatment options but did not evaluate oral versus intravenous antiviral treatment.

Intravitreal concentrations of valacyclovir attain inhibitory concentrations against VZV, HSV-1, and HSV-2 [32]. The ocular penetration of valacyclovir is up to 25% of serum concentration [32] and achieves the reported inhibitory ranges for drug level for inhibition of VZV, HSV-1, and HSV-2. Simulation models demonstrate that high-dose valacyclovir reaches comparable vitreous drug concentration as intravenous acyclovir [33]. Valacyclovir is preferred over oral acyclovir due to its superior pharmacokinetic characteristics. It has excellent bioavailability of up to 54.2% [34]. Oral valacyclovir achieves three to five times higher plasma levels than oral acyclovir. (Weller). In patients who are unreliable with medication compliance, or present with bilateral viral retinitis, hospital admission for intravenous antivirals is reasonable. In contrast, oral acyclovir does not demonstrate the vitreous penetration that its prodrug valacyclovir can achieve. PORN generally requires higher doses of antiviral medication and has a worse prognosis [35]. This is usually managed with systemic antivirals plus intravitreal injections. Valacyclovir is dosed at 500 mg three times daily for HSV and 1 g three times daily for VZV, although many specialists will use the 1 gram dose for extensive retinal necrosis regardless of etiologic virus to attain high vitreous concentration of antiviral. Given the potential for rapid vision decline, some specialists recommend an initial dose of 2 g three times daily for at least 3 weeks or until areas of retinitis begin to pigment at the edges. Subsequently, valacyclovir dosing can be reduced to 1 g daily for maintenance, with most practitioners recommending lifetime prophylaxis to prevent reactivation or involvement of the fellow eye.

Important adverse effects of systemic antivirals include thrombotic thrombocytopenic purpura/hemolytic uremic syndrome (TTP/HUS) and nephrotoxicity, so its use is contraindicated with patients with certain pre-existing hematologic abnormalities. Baseline comprehensive metabolic panel should be obtained prior to or at the time of medication initiation, as dose adjustments should be made based on renal function.

Adjunctive therapy with intravitreal foscarnet has been shown to reduce the risk of retinal detachment compared to systemic therapy alone [25, 36]. Patients receiving combination therapy instead of systemic therapy alone were also more likely to gain two or more lines of visual acuity [36]. Additionally, intravitreal therapy represents an important treatment modality in situations in which there are contraindications to or dosing restrictions of systemic treatment, most commonly related to acute or chronic renal dysfunction.

Acyclovir resistance in HSV has an incidence of roughly 0.1–0.7% [35]. Such resistance in VZV is significantly lower but not well defined. Acyclovir resistance is mediated by mutations in viral thymidine kinase which inhibits phosphorylation of the antiviral into its active form. The common genes associated with this are UL23 in HSV or ORF36 in VZV. Resistance should be suspected in patients who have been on long-term suppressive therapy and present with a breakthrough infection or fail to respond in a reasonable time frame to appropriately dosed antiviral therapy. If acyclovir resistance is suspected, foscarnet is the alternative agent of choice due to low cross-resistance between the two classes of antivirals [35].

In patients who develop secondary retinal detachment during the cicatricial phase, surgical repair is successful, and there is no difference in rate of recurrent RD with pars plana vitrectomy versus combined pars plana vitrectomy with scleral buckle [37]. There is a high rate of re-detachment after initial retinal detachment repair, with 6 of 13 eyes having developed recurrent retinal detachment within the first postoperative year in one series by Kopplin et al. [37].

Some practitioners have advocated for the use of prophylactic laser retinopexy to prevent retinal detachment during the cicatricial phase. However, studies assessing outcomes are limited by selection bias, as laser retinopexy requires relatively clearer media and those patients tended to have better starting visual acuity and lesser degree of retinitis involvement [27]. The American Academy of Ophthalmology does not specifically recommend this practice due to insufficient evidence to conclude a benefit [27].

Early vitrectomy prior to retinal detachment has also been proposed as another prophylactic treatment to improve long-term visual outcomes. Potential benefits include removal of inflammatory mediators in the vitreous cavity, removal of tractional membranes, application of prophylactic laser, and placement of long-term tamponade [27]. Studies show mixed results of visual and anatomic benefit, and the American Academy of Ophthalmology found insufficient evidence to conclude whether benefit existed. Intervention prior to the lifting of the hyaloid face in patients without pre-existing PVD can be considered, as hyaloidal traction is a likely inciting factor of retinal detachment in many of these cases.

Commonly, HSV and VZV retinitis will appear to worsen slightly following the initiation of therapy; this is likely due to greater involvement of the retina than is visualized on initial exam. In a natural history study of ARN, progression of retinal lesions was occasionally observed within the first 48 hours, and regression was observed a mean 3.9 days after initiation of antiviral therapy. It is also common to see an inflammatory response, such as progression of vitritis, following initiation of therapy, which has been speculated to reflect immunologic mechanisms rather than infectious progression [38]. With treatment, the areas of retinal whitening will pigment at the edges first, following a centripetal pattern.

The anticipated visual prognosis of HSV/VZV retinitis is dependent upon the degree and location of retinitis noted at presentation, as well as other associated ocular findings. There is a correlation between the extent of retinal involvement and worse visual outcome [39], and retinitis involving the macula was a common etiology of visual acuity worse than 20/40 [38]. Retinal arterial sheathing, sclerosis, and dye leakage on fluorescein angiography in a diffuse pattern extending from the optic nerve (rather than limited to areas of peripheral retinal involvement) are associated with poor visual prognosis [40], as they can lead to secondary ischemic optic neuropathy or large areas of retinal hypoxia. Optic nerve dysfunction, which can clinically present as an edematous or pale optic disc, can be ischemic or infiltrative (by immune cells) [38, 41]. It is also associated with worse visual acuity outcomes and is common in eyes with greater than 50% retinal involvement [38, 39]. Finally, retinal detachment is a significant cause of vision loss following ARN [38, 39].

CMV Retinitis

CMV retinitis has historically required inpatient admission for induction therapy with intravenous ganciclovir 5 mg/kg twice daily, with subsequent transition to oral maintenance therapy. First-line induction therapy is oral valganciclovir 900 mg twice daily for 3 weeks. Multiple recent studies have demonstrated that valganciclovir achieves comparable plasma drug levels and area under curve compared to intravenous ganciclovir [42]. There was no difference in relative risk of retinitis progression with valganciclovir compared to intravenous ganciclovir induction [42]. Additionally, valganciclovir is cost-effective compared to traditional intravenous induction regimens due to costs associated with inpatient admission and management of complications associated with intravenous drug administration or prolonged hospital stay [43].

Antiviral resistance is more common in CMV than in HSV or VZV and can occur through multiple known mutations including UL54 mutations which instill resistance to ganciclovir, valganciclovir, foscarnet, and cidofovir. Letermovir resistance can occur with UL56, UL51, or UL89 mutations. Maribavir resistance can develop through UL97 kinase mutations [44]. Resistance and disease progression are associated with plasma CMV viral load above 400 international units in spite of therapy, persistent retinitis in spite of the use of a ganciclovir implant, breakthrough infections that occur on chemoprophylaxis, or failure of infection to respond clinically in a reasonable time frame [13]. Of note, immune reconstitution inflammatory syndrome (IRIS) following initiation of antiretroviral therapy in HIV patients with CMV retinitis can mimic worsening of retinitis without true antiviral resistance [14, 45]. The incidence of immune recovery uveitis is estimated to be around 0.1 per person-year and is typically associated with cystoid macular edema, epiretinal membrane formation, and neovascularization of the disc [46]. Patients with larger areas of CMV retinitis involvement are at greater risk for the development of immune recovery uveitis [47].

Adverse effects of valganciclovir include the risk of myelosuppression and nephrotoxicity, which can limit its use in some patients.

The intravitreal ganciclovir implant (Vitrasert, B&L) was previously used for the treatment of CMV retinitis during the era of HIV/AIDS prior to the advent of modern-day antiretroviral therapy. The implant is placed surgically and releases 1mcg/hr over a period of 5 to 8 months [48]. It was shown to slow time to progression in the affected eye [49]; however, local therapy with the implant alone was associated with contralateral eye involvement and systemic disease [13, 50]. Systemic therapy is superior to intraocular therapy in reducing mortality, incidence of visceral CMV disease, and contralateral eye involvement [13, 50]. Despite the relative superiority of systemic therapy in reducing contralateral eye involvement in HIV patients, the risk remains 26.1% per person-year, which is still considerable [51]. Reported ocular complications associated with the ganciclovir implant include cataract formation, vitreous hemorrhage, retinal detachment, endophthalmitis, and epiretinal membrane formation [52, 53]. The implant was discontinued in 2013 due to declining incidence of CMV retinitis in the setting of improved systemic therapeutics for HIV/AIDS.

Intravitreal foscarnet (2.4 mg/0.1 mL) is a useful intravitreal agent at the time of clinical diagnosis while awaiting molecular confirmation, due to its efficacy against VZV, HSV-1,2, and CMV. Intravitreal ganciclovir (2 mg/0.1 mL) and cidofovir (20 mg/0.1 mL), in contrast, are solely effective against CMV retinitis, but may be administered in patients with CMV-positive aqueous PCR as monotherapy or adjunctive therapy, specifically with contraindications to or dose restrictions of systemic therapy or sight-threatening lesions. Due to lack of widespread availability of intravitreal foscarnet, intravitreal ganciclovir is sometimes used for non-CMV retinitis, but should be used only in conjunction with systemic valacyclovir therapy for adequate coverage. Due to the relatively short half-life, twice weekly injections are recommended initially and can be spaced out as retinal lesions begin to pigment.

Other FDA-approved therapies for CMV retinitis include intravenous foscarnet or cidofovir, both of which are associated with nephrotoxicity that can limit systemic administration in patients with underlying renal dysfunction [54]. Fomivirsen (intravitreal) is also FDA-approved as a second-therapy; because it is only available intravitreally, there is minimal systemic absorption and minimal systemic side effects [54]. However, as with the ganciclovir implant, it was withdrawn from market due to decreased demand for intravitreal CMV therapy with improved control of HIV/AIDS.

For patients with HIV infection, initiation of highly active antiretroviral therapy (HAART) is indicated to address the underlying immunocompromise.

The expected course of CMV retinitis can be similar to that of HSV and VZV retinitis, with slight worsening prior to improvement. Visual prognosis of CMV retinitis is often better than that of HSV and VZV, primarily due to the fact that CMV retinitis is more commonly localized to one quadrant and progresses at a slower rate [55]. However, in cases with optic nerve involvement or extensive retinitis at presentation, prognosis can be poor. Similar to HSV and VZV retinitis, retinal lesions in CMV responding to therapy should pigment at the edges and move centrally. Many practitioners advise patients to remain on lifelong antiviral prophylaxis in the absence of any contraindications. In cases of CMV retinitis, if the underlying risk factor was reversible immunocompromise such as untreated HIV infection/AIDS, antiviral prophylaxis can be discontinued after reconstitution of sufficient T-cell count with HAART [56, 57].

Cases

Case 1: VZV Acute Retinal Necrosis

A 77-year-old Caucasian woman presented for 3-week history of blurred vision in the left eye. She had been initially treated with tobramycin eye drops for redness and irritation without benefit. Her medical history was significant for rheumatoid arthritis, for which she was being treated with prednisone 10 mg daily and methotrexate 12.5 mg weekly, and two prior shingles episodes involving the right forehead and back of the neck. The rest of her medical history was noncontributory. On exam, her BCVA was 20/25 and 20/40, and IOP was 8 and 10 in the right and left eyes, respectively. Anterior slit lamp examination revealed a quiet anterior chamber and vitreous cavity and early cataracts. Dilated fundoscopic exam revealed confluent peripheral retinal whitening in the left eye, with multifocal patches of retinal whitening and few intraretinal hemorrhages extending posteriorly without macular or optic disc involvement and extensive retinal arteriolar sclerosis (Fig. 5.1). Optical coherence tomography (OCT) demonstrated pre-retinal opacities and outer retinal changes (Fig. 5.2). An anterior chamber paracentesis was performed, and aqueous fluid was sent for VZV, HSV, CMV, and Toxoplasma PCR. Intravitreal foscarnet 2.4 mg/0.1 ml was administered, and the patient was started on valganciclovir 2 mg three times daily. The aqueous sample tested positive for VZV by PCR. The patient was re-examined 2 days later with slight progression of retinitis. However, the retinitis stabilized and then began to pigment at the borders with continued foscarnet injections. The patient received biweekly

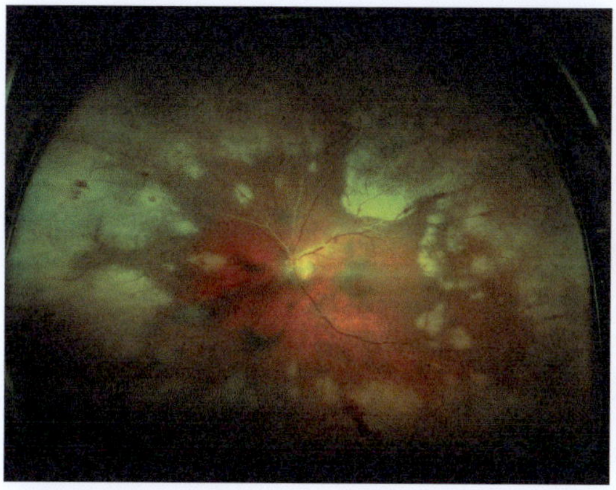

Fig. 5.1 Wide-field fundus photo of active phase of acute retinal necrosis

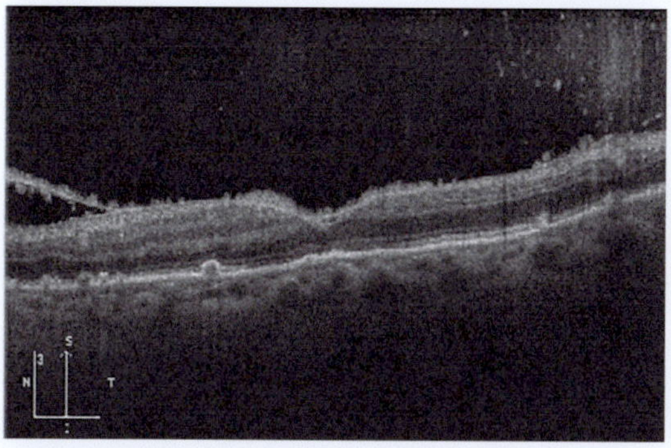

Fig. 5.2 OCT of acute retinal necrosis

intravitreal foscarnet for total of four doses, after which it was reduced to once weekly once pigmentation was observed at multiple lesion borders. Injections were stopped once all borders of retinitis appeared fully pigmented. The patient was also initially started on topical prednisolone eyedrops and oral prednisone 20 mg daily for an expected increase in anterior chamber and vitreous cell around 2 weeks after initial presentation. Steroid therapy in conjunction with local and systemic antiviral therapy led to clinical improvement. Three months later, exam and imaging showed resolution of active retinitis with residual peripheral retinal atrophy and proliferative vitreoretinopathy without retinal detachment (Figs. 5.3 and 5.4).

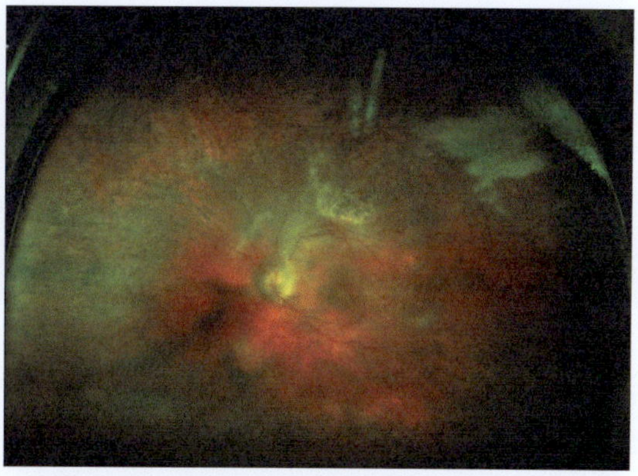

Fig. 5.3 Resolved acute retinal necrosis with proliferative vitreoretinopathy (cicatricial phase)

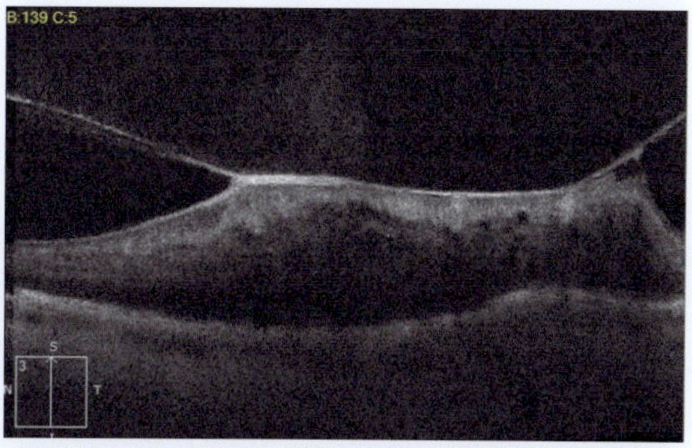

Fig. 5.4 OCT of proliferative vitreoretinopathy (cicatricial phase)

Case 2: CMV Retinitis

A 58-year-old African man presented with right eye pain and vision loss. His medical history included Type 1 diabetes mellitus and pulmonary sarcoidosis. One week prior to referral, he had been diagnosed with iritis by an outside practitioner and started on prednisolone and cyclopentolate. Right eye visual acuity was 20/125, decreased from 1 week prior. Slit lamp exam revealed extensive keratic precipitates and both anterior chamber and vitreous cells in the right eye. Fundoscopic exam demonstrated vascular sheathing and multiple areas of retinitis bilaterally, right eye worse than left (Fig. 5.5a, b). His

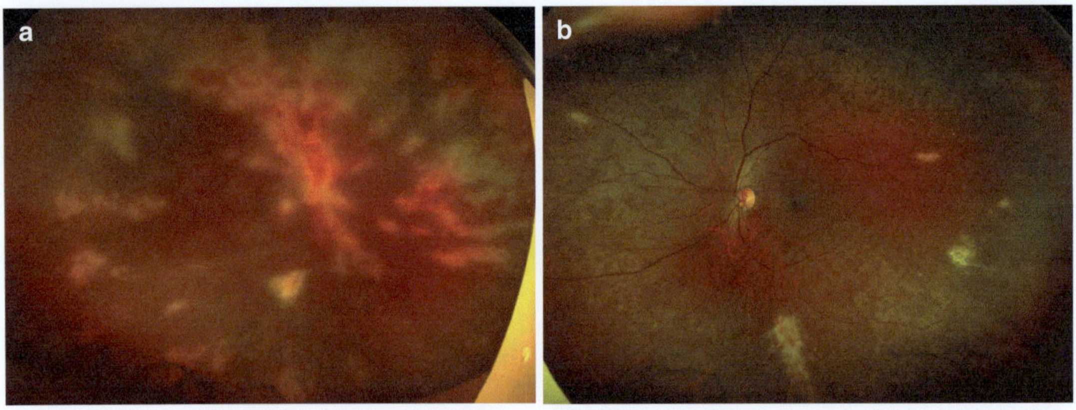

Fig. 5.5 (**a**, **b**) Bilateral CMV retinitis, with asymmetric involvement of right eye

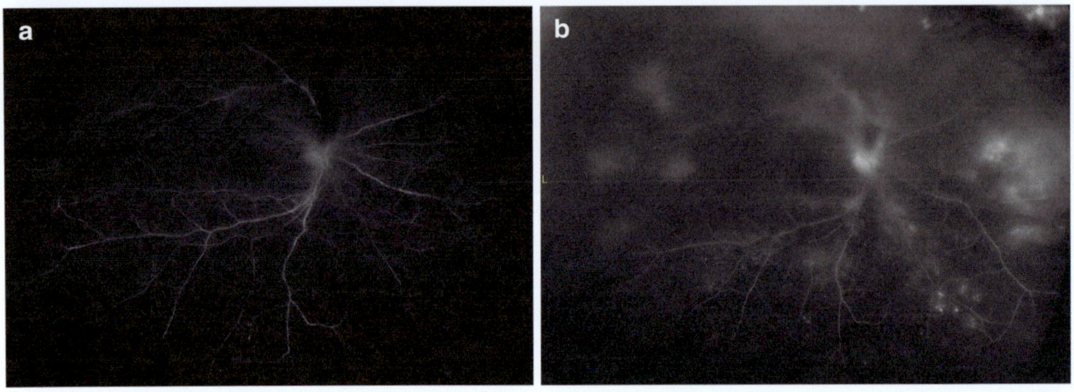

Fig. 5.6 (**a**, **b**) Fluorescein angiography of CMV retinitis, right eye. (**a**) Early frames demonstrate areas of nonperfusion and leakage against background of diabetic retinopathy. (**b**) Late frames show progressive leakage from areas of retinitis and nerve, some blockage by areas of intraretinal hemorrhage

exam also demonstrated right optic disc elevation. Fluorescein angiography demonstrated retinal vascular leakage (Fig. 5.6a, b). An anterior chamber tap was performed, and the patient received intravitreal foscarnet 2.4 mg/0.1 mL in both eyes. He was empirically started on valacyclovir 2 g three times a day, and prednisolone was increased to hourly. The aqueous sample was submitted for PCR for CMV, HSV, VZV, and toxoplasma, in addition to serological testing for HIV, syphilis, and tuberculosis, and to assess baseline hematological, renal, and hepatic status. His aqueous sample PCR was positive for the presence of CMV, and his lab results led to a new diagnosis of HIV infection. He was referred to infectious diseases and started on highly active antiretroviral therapy (elvitegravir, cobicistat, emtricitabine, and tenofovir). He was switched from valacyclovir to valganciclovir 900 mg twice daily, with plans for monitoring via weekly complete blood count. He was treated with twice weekly intravitreal foscarnet injection initially and then decreased to once weekly injections until resolution of active retinitis. As his retinitis improved, prednisolone was weaned to once daily, and valganciclovir was decreased to 900 mg daily.

Six months after initial presentation, he was noted to have bilateral recurrence of CMV retinitis. At that time the infectious diseases specialist recommended a course of intravenous ganciclovir 5 mg/kg twice daily via a peripherally inserted central catheter (PICC line). A repeat aqueous paracentesis was performed which confirmed persistence of CMV intraocularly. He received adjunctive intravitreal foscarnet in addition to IV ganciclovir. The active retinitis resolved in the right eye and improved substantially in the left eye, and he was transitioned back to oral valganciclovir 900 mg twice daily after 6 weeks. Due to his protracted course, there was suspicion of ganciclovir resistance, but insufficient quantity of aqueous humor could be obtained for susceptibility testing. A small amount of active retinitis persisted in the left eye.

Around 9 months after initial presentation, the patient developed a new right rhegmatogenous retinal detachment with subretinal fluid encroaching into inferior macula beyond the arcades. He underwent repair with combined pars plana vitrectomy with silicone oil and scleral buckle of the right eye.

Conflicts of Interest The authors attest they have no relevant conflicts of interest to the material discussed.

References

1. Lancini D, Faddy HM, Flower R, Hogan C. Cytomegalovirus disease in immunocompetent adults. Med J Aust. 2014;201(10):578–80.
2. Fatahzadeh M, Schwartz RA. Human herpes simplex virus infections: Epidemiology, pathogenesis, symptomatology, diagnosis, and management. J Am Acad Dermatol. 2007;57(5):737–63.
3. Balasopoulou A, Kokkinos P, Pagoulatos D, Plotas P, Makri OE, Georgakopoulos CD, et al. Post-fever retinitis- Newer concepts. BMC Ophthalmol. 2017;17(1):1.
4. Salceanu SO, Raman V. Recurrent chikungunya retinitis. BMJ Case Rep. 2018;2018:1–4.
5. Konjevoda S, Dzelalija B, Canovic S, Pastar Z, Savic V, Tabain I, et al. West nile virus retinitis in a patient with neuroinvasive disease. Rev. Soc Bras Med Trop. 2019;52(March):0–2.
6. Steiner I. Herpes virus infection of the peripheral nervous system [Internet]. In: Handbook of Clinical Neurology, vol. 115. first ed. Elsevier B.V; 2013. p. 543–58. https://doi.org/10.1016/B978-0-444-52902-2.00031-X.
7. Centers for Disease Control and Prevention (CDC). Varicella incidence. MMWR Morb Mortal Wkly Rep. 2012;61(12):201–4.
8. Ritterband DC, Friedberg DN. Virus infections of the eye. Rev. Med Virol. 1998;8(4):187–201.
9. Farooq AV, Valyi-Nagy T, Shukla D. Mediators and mechanisms of herpes simplex virus entry into ocular cells. Curr Eye Res. 2010;35(6):445–50.
10. Tiwari V, Oh M, Kovacs M. Role for nectin-1 in herpes simplex virus 1 entry and spread in human retinal pigment epithelial cells. Bone [Internet]. 2014;23(1):1–7. Available from: https://www.ncbi.nlm.nih.gov/pmc/articles/PMC3624763/pdf/nihms412728.pdf
11. Au Eong KG, Beatty S, Charles SJ. Cytomegalovirus retinitis in patients with acquired immune deficiency syndrome. Postgrad Med J. 1999;75(888):585–90.
12. Kim JY, Hong SY, Park WK, Kim RY, Kim M, Park YG, et al. Prognostic factors of cytomegalovirus retinitis after hematopoietic stem cell transplantation. PLoS One [Internet]. 2020;15(9):1–13. https://doi.org/10.1371/journal.pone.0238257.
13. Jabs DA, Martin BK, Forman MS, Ricks MO. Erratum: Cytomegalovirus (CMV) blood DNA load, CMV retinitis progression, and occurrence of resistant CMV in patients with CMV retinitis (Journal of Infectious Diseases (August 15, 2005) 192 (640–649)). J Infect Dis. 2005;192(7):1310.
14. Jabs DA, Van Nattta K, Holland G, Danis R. Cytomegalovirus retinitis in patients with AIDS after initiating antiretroviral therapy. Am J Ophthalmol. 2017;174:e761–7.
15. Deliège PG, Bastien J, Mokri L, Guyot-Colosio C, Arndt C, Rieu P. Belatacept associated - cytomegalovirus retinitis in a kidney transplant recipient: a case report and review of the literature. BMC Ophthalmol. 2020;20(1):1–5.
16. Camargo JF, Komanduri KV. Emerging concepts in cytomegalovirus infection following hematopoietic stem cell transplantation. Hematol Oncol Stem Cell Ther [Internet]. 2017;10(4):233–8. https://doi.org/10.1016/j.hemonc.2017.05.001.
17. Son G, Lee JY, Kim JG, Kim YJ. Clinical features of cytomegalovirus retinitis after solid organ transplantation versus hematopoietic stem cell transplantation. Graefe's Arch Clin Exp Ophthalmol. 2020;259(3):585–91.
18. Rao NA, Zhang J, Ishimoto SI, Jabs DA, Green WR, Pulido J. Role of retinal vascular endothelial cells in development of CMV retinitis. Trans Am Ophthalmol Soc. 1998;96:111–26.
19. Pereira L, Maidji E, Tugizov SJT. Deletion mutants in human cytomegalovirus glycoprotein US9 are impaired in cell-cell transmission and in altering tight junctions of polarized human retinal pigment epithelial cells. Scand J Infect Dis Suppl. 1995;99:82–7.
20. Scholz M, Doerr HWCJ. Human cytomegalovirus retinitis: pathogenicity, immune evasion and persistence. Trends Microbiol. 2003;11(4):171–8.
21. Davis JL, Solomon D, Nussenblatt RB, Palestine AG, Chan CC. Immunocytochemical staining of vitreous cells: indications, techniques, and results. Ophthalmology [Internet]. 1992;99(2):250–6. https://doi.org/10.1016/S0161-6420(92)31984-0.

22. Holland GN. Standard diagnostic criteria for the acute retinal necrosis syndrome. Am J Ophthalmol. 1994;117(5):663–6.
23. Kianersi F, Masjedi A, Ghanbari H. Acute retinal necrosis after herpetic encephalitis. Case Rep Ophthalmol. 2010;1(2):85–9.
24. Austin RB. Progressive outer retinal necrosis syndrome: A comprehensive review of its clinical presentation, relationship to immune system status, and management. Clin Eye Vis Care. 2000;12(3–4):119–29.
25. Wong R, Pavesio CE, Laidlaw DAH, Williamson TH, Graham EM, Stanford MR. Acute retinal necrosis. the effects of intravitreal foscarnet and virus type on outcome. Ophthalmology [Internet]. 2010;117(3):556–60. https://doi.org/10.1016/j.ophtha.2009.08.003.
26. Miller JM, Binnicker MJ, Campbell S, Carroll KC, Chapin KC, Gilligan PH, et al. A guide to utilization of the microbiology laboratory for diagnosis of infectious diseases: 2018 update by the infectious diseases society of America and the American society for microbiology. Clin Infect Dis. 2018;67(6):e1–94.
27. Schoenberger SD, Kim SJ, Thorne JE, Mruthyunjaya P, Yeh S, Bakri SJ, et al. Diagnosis and treatment of acute retinal necrosis: a report by the american academy of ophthalmology. Ophthalmology [Internet]. 2017;124(3):382–92. https://doi.org/10.1016/j.ophtha.2016.11.007.
28. Tran THC, Rozenberg F, Cassoux N, Rao NA, LeHoang P, Bodaghi B. Polymerase chain reaction analysis of aqueous humour samples in necrotising retinitis. Br J Ophthalmol. 2003;87(1):79–83.
29. Aizman A, Johnson MW, Elner SG. Treatment of acute retinal necrosis syndrome with oral antiviral medications. Ophthalmology. 2007;114(2):307–12.
30. Emerson GG, Smith JR, Wilson DJ, Rosenbaum JT, Flaxel CJ. Primary treatment of acute retinal necrosis with oral antiviral therapy. Ophthalmology. 2006;113(12):2259–61.
31. Zhao X, Meng L, Zhang W, Wang D, Chen Y. Retinal detachment following acute retinal necrosis and the efficacies of different interventions. Vol. Publish Ah, Retina. 2020.
32. Huynh TH, Johnson MW, Comer GM, Fish DN. Vitreous penetration of orally administered valacyclovir. Am J Ophthalmol. 2008;145(4):682–6.
33. Liu T, Jain A, Fung M. valacyclovir as initial treatment for acute retinal necrosis: a pharmacokinetic modeling and simulation study. Physiol Behav. 2017;176(3):139–48.
34. Jacobson MA, Gallant J, Wang LH, Coakley D, Weller S, Gary D, et al. Phase I trial of valaciclovir, the L-valyl ester of acyclovir, in patients with advanced human immunodeficiency virus disease. Antimicrob Agents Chemother. 1994;38(7):1534–40.
35. Piret J, Boivin G. Antiviral resistance in herpes simplex virus and varicella-zoster virus infections: Diagnosis and management. Curr Opin Infect Dis. 2016;29(6):654–62.
36. Yeh S, Suhler EB, Smith JR, Bruce B, Fahle G, Bailey ST, Hwang TS, Stout JT, Lauer AK, Wilson DJ, Rosenbaum JT, et al. Combination systemic and intravitreal antiviral therapy in the management of acute retinal necrosis syndrome. Ophthalmic Surg Lasers Imaging Retin. 2014;45(5):399–407.
37. Kopplin LJ, Thomas AS, Cramer S, Kim YH, Yeh S, Lauer AKFC. Long-Term Surgical Outcomes of Retinal Detachment Associated With Acute Retinal Necrosis. Ophthalmic Surg Lasers Imaging Retin. 2016;47(7):660–4.
38. Blumenkranz MS, Culbertson WW, Clarkson JG, Dix R. Treatment of the Acute Retinal Necrosis Syndrome with Intravenous Acyclovir. Ophthalmology [Internet]. 1986;93(3):296–300. https://doi.org/10.1016/S0161-6420(86)33740-0.
39. Meghpara B, Sulkowski G, Kesen MR, Tessler HH, Goldstein DA. Long-term follow-up of acute retinal necrosis. Retina. 2010;30(5):795–800.
40. Matsuo T, Morimoto K, Matsuo N. Factors associated with poor visual outcome in acute retinal necrosis. Br J Ophthalmol. 1991;75(8):450–4.
41. Chang S, Young LH. Acute retinal necrosis: An overview. Int Ophthalmol Clin. 2007;47(2):145–54.
42. Martin D, Sierra-Madero J. a Controlled Trial of Valganciclovir As Induction Therapy for Cytomegalovirus Retinitis. Infect Dis Clin Pract. 2002;11(3):180–1.
43. Somerville K. Cost advantages of oral drug therapy for managing cytomegalovirus disease. Control Commun Dis Man. 2015;60:9–12.
44. Hakki M. Moving Past Ganciclovir and Foscarnet: Advances in CMV Therapy. Curr Hematol Malig Rep. 2020;15(2):90–102.
45. Heiden D, Tun N, Smithuis FN, Keenan JD, Oldenburg CE, Holland GN, et al. Active cytomegalovirus retinitis after the start of antiretroviral therapy. Br J Ophthalmol. 2019;103(2):157–60.
46. Nguyen QD, Kempen J, Bolton S, Dunn J, Jabs D. Immune Recovery Uveitis in Patients With. 2000;9394(00):634–9.
47. Karavellas MP, Azen SP, MacDonald JC, Shufelt CL, Lowder CY, Plummer DJ, et al. Immune recovery vitritis and uveitis in aids: Clinical predictors, sequelae, and treatment outcomes. Retina. 2001;21(1):1–9.
48. Wang J, Jiang A, Joshi M, Christoforidis J. Drug delivery implants in the treatment of vitreous inflammation. Mediators Inflamm. 2013;2013:780634.
49. Martin DF, Parks DJ, Mellow SD, Ferris FL, Walton C, Remaley NA, et al. Treatment of intraocular sustained-release ganciclovir cytomegalovirus retinitis with a sustained-release ganciclovir implant. N Engl J Med. 1997;337(2):83–90.
50. Murray J, Hilbig A, Soe TT, Ei WLSS, Soe KP, Ciglenecki I. Treating HIV-associated cytomegalovirus retinitis with oral valganciclovir and intra-ocular ganciclovir by primary HIV clinicians in southern Myanmar: a retrospective analysis of routinely collected data. BMC Infect Dis. 2020;20(1):1–8.

51. Kempen JH, Jabs DA, Wilson LA, Dunn JP, West SK. Incidence of cytomegalovirus (CMV) retinitis in second eyes of patients with the acquired immune deficiency syndrome and unilateral CMV retinitis. Am J Ophthalmol. 2005;139(6):1028–34.
52. Shane TS, Martin DF. Endophthalmitis after ganciclovir implant in patients with AIDS and cytomegalovirus retinitis. Am J Ophthalmol. 2003;136(4):649–54.
53. Lim JI, Wolitz RA, Dowling AH, Bloom HR, Irvine AR, Schwartz DM. Visual and anatomic outcomes associated with posterior segment complications after ganciclovir implant procedures in patients with AIDS and cytomegalovirus retinitis. Am J Ophthalmol. 1999;127(3):288–93.
54. Biron KK. Antiviral drugs for cytomegalovirus diseases. Antiviral Res. 2006;71(2–3):154–63.
55. Patel A, Young L. CMV retinitis. In: Uveitis. 2017:45–52.
56. Jouan M, Savès M, Tubiana R, Carcelain G, Cassoux N, Aubron-Olivier C, et al. Discontinuation of maintenance therapy for cytomegalovirus retinitis in HIV-infected patients receiving highly active antiretroviral therapy. Aids. 2001;15(1):23–31.
57. Berenguer J, Gonzaález J, Pulido F, Padilla B, Casado JL, Rubio R, et al. Discontinuation of secondary prophylaxis in patients with cytomegalovirus retinitis who have responded to highly active antiretroviral therapy. Clin Infect Dis. 2002;34(3):394–7.

Vector-Borne Infections

6

Sara L. Hojjatie, Steven Yeh, Jessica G. Shantha, Lucileia Teixeira, and John L. Johnson

Abbreviations

BBB	blood-brain barrier
BRB	blood-retinal barrier
CHIKV	Chikungunya virus
CWS	cotton wool spots
DENV1, DENV2, DENV3, DENV4	dengue fever virus 1, 2, 3, and 4
ELISA	enzyme-linked immunosorbent assays
MAC-ELISA	IgM antibody-capture enzyme-linked immunosorbent assay
NAAT	nucleic acid amplification testing
NSAIDs	nonsteroidal anti-inflammatory drugs
RNA	ribonuclear virus
RNFL	retinal nerve fiber layer
RPE	retinal pigment epithelium
RT-PCR	reverse transcriptase polymerase chain reaction
WNV	West Nile virus

S. L. Hojjatie
Department of Ophthalmology, University of Washington, Seattle, WA, USA
e-mail: shojjat@uw.edu

S. Yeh (✉)
Department of Ophthalmology, Emory University, Atlanta, GA, USA

Truhlsen Eye Institute, University of Nebraska Medical Center, Omaha, NE, USA
e-mail: Steven.yeh@emory.edu

J. G. Shantha
Department of Ophthalmology, Emory University, Atlanta, GA, USA

Francis I. Proctor Foundation for Research in Ophthalmology, University of California San Francisco, San Francisco, CA, USA
e-mail: jshanth@emory.edu

L. Teixe ira
Department of Infectious Diseases, Cleveland Clinic, Cleveland, OH, USA
e-mail: johnsol12@ccf.org

J. L. Johnson
Department of Medicine and Global Health and Diseases, Case Western Reserve University School of Medicine and University Hospitals Cleveland Medical Center, Cleveland, OH, USA
e-mail: jlj@case.edu

Introduction

Arboviruses are a leading cause of systemic human infections worldwide [1]. These viruses are transmitted by biting arthropod vectors, such as the *Aedes aegypti* and *A. albopictus* mosquitoes, as well as ticks [1]. Diseases caused by arboviruses including dengue, Zika, Chikungunya, yellow fever, and West Nile are important causes of morbidity and mortality worldwide. Dengue fever alone affects more than 390 million people every year in tropical and subtropical areas of the world [2]. Arbovirus infections occur most frequently in the tropics; their recent spread into temperate areas may be explained

© Springer Nature Switzerland AG 2023
C. Y. Lowder et al. (eds.), *Emerging Ocular Infections*, Essentials in Ophthalmology,
https://doi.org/10.1007/978-3-031-24559-6_6

by the expansion of *Aedes* mosquito populations in those areas [3]. The ability of vectors to bridge spatial and ecologic gaps between animals and humans has led to massive global epidemics of arboviral infections in recent years—as exemplified by large outbreaks in the Americas of dengue fever in the 1990s, West Nile virus in the 2000s, and Chikungunya and Zika viruses in 2015 [4].

In humans, symptoms of arbovirus disease generally occur 3 to 15 days after infection and last 3 or 4 days. The most frequent symptoms are rash, fever, malaise, headache, myalgia, and arthralgia. Therapy for arboviral diseases is supportive. Prevention, including public measures to reduce the number of vectors and personal protection, remains the mainstay for arthropod vector-borne disease control.

Ocular manifestations of arboviruses are uncommon due to under-reporting [1]. The most common ocular presentations include conjunctivitis, uveitis, as well as posterior segment disease such as choroiditis, chorioretinal atrophy, and retinitis [1]. The goal of this chapter is to describe the ocular manifestations of arboviruses, including yellow fever virus (YFV), dengue virus (DENV), Zika virus (ZIKV), West Nile virus (WNV), and Chikungunya virus (CHIKV).

Pathogenesis

The eye is sequestered from systemic circulation by a blood-retinal barrier (BRB), an extension of the blood-brain barrier (BBB) [1, 4]. Disruption of the outer BRB, formed by the retinal pigment epithelium (RPE), may create a route of entry for a virus. However, the underlying molecular mechanism that allows for the breach of this barrier is unknown [1, 3, 4].

Virology and Diagnosis of Arboviral Infections

Dengue, West Nile, and Zika viruses are flaviviruses with similar transmission cycles. Chikungunya is an alphavirus. Alphaviruses and flaviviruses are enveloped positive-sense single-stranded RNA viruses. Laboratory diagnosis of arboviral infection depends upon detection of the viral genome in the blood by reverse transcriptase polymerase chain reaction (RT-PCR) during the first few days after symptoms appear. PCR tests become positive during the viremic phase: from the first through the sixth day. For patients with suspected dengue or Zika virus disease, nucleic acid amplification tests (NAATs) are the preferred method of diagnosis because they provide confirmed evidence of infection and identify the specific virus causing the infection [5]. Immunoglobulin M (IgM) and neutralizing antibody testing also can be used to identify acute viral infections, particularly in patients who present after viral nucleic acid is no longer detectable in the bloodstream [5–7]. RT-PCR in serum is the main test for ZIKV, CHIKV, WNV, and DENV during the initial viremic phase. Detection of ZIKV RNA in serum is limited to the first 5 days and in urine up to 20 days. Laboratory diagnosis of Zika virus infection is challenging because of low viremia and cross-reactivity of ZIKV antibodies with other flaviviruses [8].

Clinical Features

Yellow Fever

Yellow fever, the first-described hemorrhagic fever, is a lethal arboviral disease. It is characterized by severe hepatic and renal injury, hemorrhage, and high mortality in its most fulminant form [9]. It resides in the tropical regions of Africa and South America [10]. The three types of transmission cycles, sylvatic, urban, and savanna, are important for implementing disease control [1]. Diagnosis is confirmed with serology or detection of viral RNA or antigens in blood.

Clinical manifestations of yellow fever viral infection follow a 3- to 6-day incubation period [11]. The acute febrile phase is characterized by fever, chills, malaise, headache, and generalized myalgia, usually resolving within 1 week. Approximately 75% to 85% will abort their infection and recover without developing classic yellow fever [9]. The remaining patients will progress to the toxic and often fatal phase of the disease, involving jaundice, renal failure, and hemorrhage [9]. No specific antiviral treatment exists for yellow fever, though a cost-effective 17D yellow fever vaccine is available for its prevention [9]. Supportive care is given to maximize tissue perfusion and reduce hemorrhagic complications [9].

There are increasing reports of ocular manifestations associated with acute yellow fever, with an increase of awareness among the ophthalmic community. Ophthalmic findings include conjunctival icterus, superficial hemorrhages, retinal nerve fiber layer (RNFL) infarcts, grayish outer retinal lesions, Roth spots, and cotton wool spots (CWS) [10–12]. Choroidal detachments and retinal vessel congestion have been reported as well [12]. The exact mechanism behind the pathogenesis of ocular disease associated with yellow fever remains unclear.

Dengue

Dengue fever, first reported in the late 1770s, is the most common mosquito-borne viral disease in humans. It is endemic in over 100 countries and affects 390 million people per year [2]. The *Aedes aegypti* mosquito is the main vector responsible for transmission [13]. This virus mainly affects the Americas, Southeast Asia, and the Western Pacific [13]. Four serotypes of dengue fever have been identified, namely, DENV1, DENV2, DENV3, and DENV4, with DENV2 considered to be the most virulent strain [14]. Diagnosis is confirmed with a positive dengue IgM test. No vaccine for dengue virus is currently available [14].

Dengue viral infections may be asymptomatic or show symptoms of a nonspecific viral syndrome [13]. After an incubation period of 4-10 days, symptoms continue for 2-7 days. Patients present with high fever and associated headache, retro-orbital pain, myalgia, and rash [13]. Dengue shock syndrome is a severe fatal form of illness that causes increased vascular permeability resulting in severe bleeding, organ impairment including liver and renal failure, fluid accumulation, and respiratory distress [13]. Treatment for dengue fever is supportive, with intervention directed toward providing antipyretic and analgesic medication and ensuring perfusion [13].

Ocular manifestations have been described with dengue fever, usually 7 days after the onset of illness [15]. Common clinical presentations include blurry vision, scotoma, hyposphagma, uveitis, and increased intraocular pressure [15]. On exam, findings of ocular dengue fever range from focal retinal hemorrhages, Roth-like spots, retinal edema, cotton wool spots, vasculitis, and optic neuritis (Fig. 6.1) [17, 18]. Many patients with ocular dengue have been observed to have maculopathy, including macular hemorrhage, arteriolar sheathing, cotton wool spots, perifoveal telangiectasia, and microaneurysms [15, 17, 18]. Scotomas have been observed to persist through at least 6 months of infection [18]. Retinal dysfunction may persist for several months [17]. The pathophysiologic mechanism of dengue fever and its effect on the eye is still unclear. The 5- to 7-day delay in onset of ocular symptoms supports an possible immune-mediated mechanism rather than direct viral infection [18, 19].

Zika Virus

Zika virus is a mosquito-transmitted flavivirus that was first isolated in the Zika forest of Uganda from a rhesus macaque in 1947. It has since spread throughout areas of Africa, Asia, and South America, affecting people in over 70 countries [1]. In light of the recent South American epidemic, Zika virus has recently been declared a public health emergency. Due to its circulation directly between *Aedes aegypti* mosquitoes and humans, it is capable of epidemic transmission. In addition to transmission by mosquitoes, Zika virus is capable of vertical transmission during pregnancy, during delivery, through sexual contact, and from blood transfusions [1].

Once infected, Zika virus has an incubation period of 3–14 days, with most patients being asymptomatic. The clinical signs of infection are mild, consisting of a flu-like illness that resolves after a few days [20]. Infected individuals typically experience fever, rash, headache, joint pain,

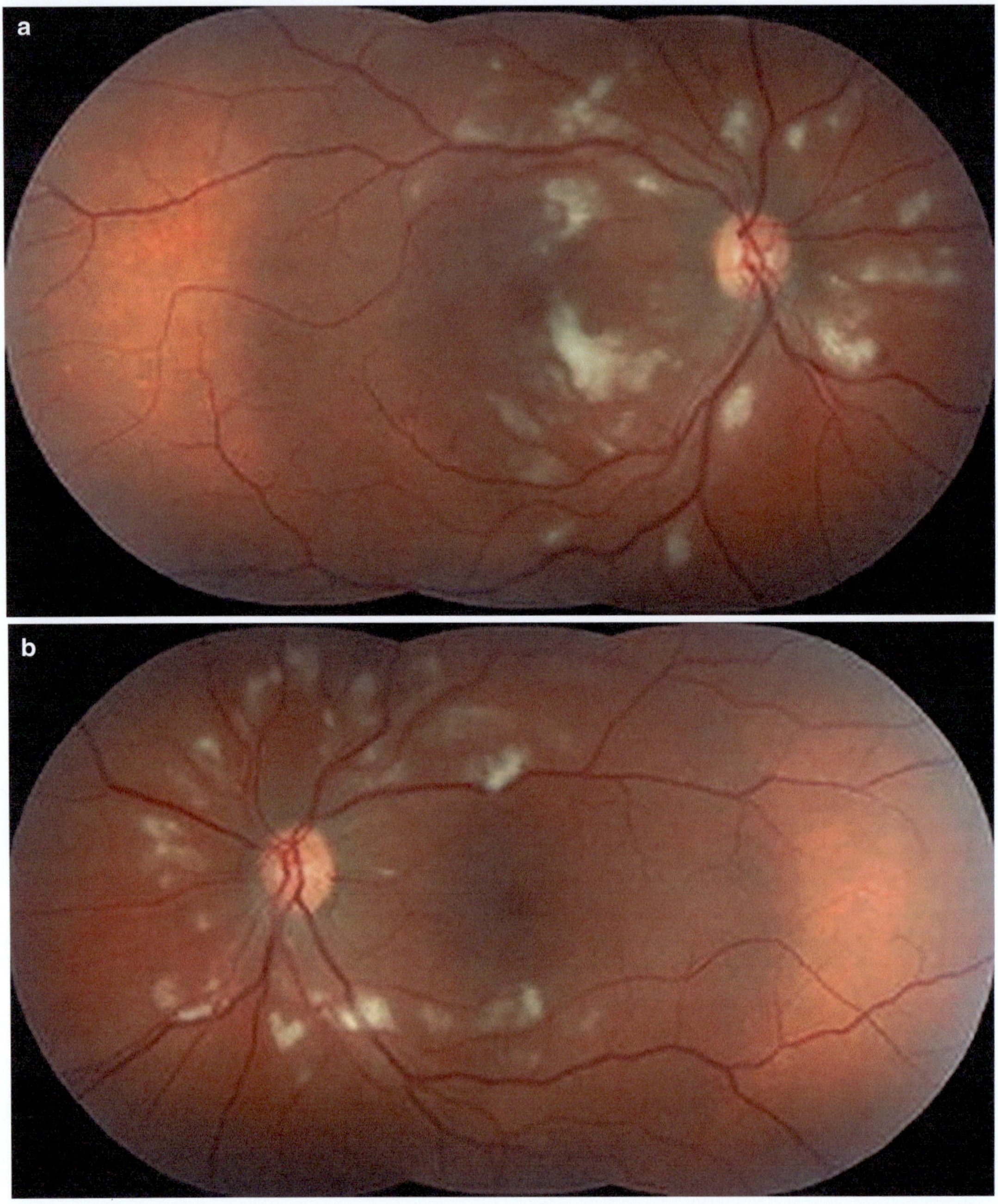

Fig. 6.1 Right (**a**) and left (**b**) eye of a patient with presumed dengue virus-related retinopathy showing retinal hemorrhage and cotton wool spots [16]. © Copyright Policy—open access. https://openi.nlm.nih.gov/

conjunctivitis, muscle pain, and possibly Guillain-Barre syndrome [21]. In severe disease, Zika virus can be associated with multi-organ failure, thrombocytopenia, and thrombocytopenic purpura. Congenital Zika virus can impair development of the fetal brain, causing microcephaly and other fetal malformations. Clinical features of congenital Zika include cerebral calcifications, hypoplasia of the cerebellum, and ventriculomegaly [20, 21].

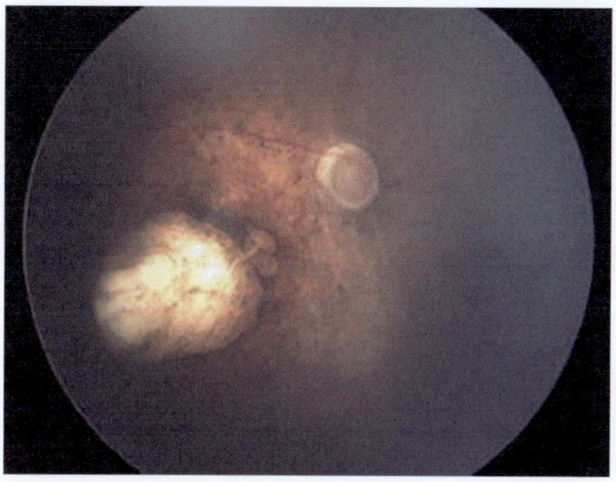

Fig. 6.2 Fundus photo of an infant with presumed Zika infection demonstrating chorioretinal scarring and pigment mottling [16]. © Copyright Policy – open access. https://openi.nlm.nih.gov/

Ocular defects are recognized as an important pathological trait of Zika virus. Zika virus commonly presents in the eye as non-purulent conjunctivitis. Additional ocular abnormalities have been described, including retinal hemorrhages, chorioretinal atrophy, posterior uveitis, optic neuritis, and maculopathies [22–26]. Due to the recent recognition of transplacental transmission, ocular manifestations of congenital Zika syndrome are of particular interest. Ocular findings in congenital Zika include macular pigment mottling, foveal reflex loss, macular neuroretinal atrophy, and fundoscopic alterations in the macular regions (Fig. 6.2) [22]. It is thought that Zika causes damage to the retina by upregulating an immune response, leading to an increase in inflammation causing retinal atrophy and cell death [23, 25, 26]. The long-term effects of Zika infection are unknown, but reports suggest that ocular lesions can be persistent [27].

West Nile Virus

West Nile virus is a neuro-invasive member of the *Flavivirus* family that was first isolated from the West Nile district of Uganda in 1937 [28]. Transmission occurs with the bite of the *Culex* mosquito, which acquires the virus after feeding on infected passerine birds. Most human infections occur between August and September. Human-to-human transmission does not occur due to the low viremia of humans, though transplacental infection and transmission through breast milk, organ donation, and blood transfusion is possible [29, 30]. Two distinct lineages of West Nile virus have been described: lineage 1, predominant in the Western world, and lineage 2, predominant in Africa. There is currently no proven treatment for West Nile virus, and therapy is supportive.

Most individuals infected with West Nile virus are asymptomatic or experience a nonspecific, mild febrile illness. The incubation period lasts between 2 and 14 days, with the self-limiting acute illness typically resolving within a week. Common symptoms of the mild illness include fevers, headache, myalgia, and gastrointestinal symptoms [28]. Other general symptoms seen in patients infected with West Nile virus include photophobia, back pain, confusion, encephalitis, and Guillain-Barre syndrome [30]. More severe presentations of the disease begin with typical West Nile fever, but later progress to mental status changes and sometimes coma [28]. A small percentage of patients experience severe neurologic disease, such as meningitis, encephalitis, or poliomyelitis [28–30].

Ophthalmic sequelae of West Nile virus have recently been recognized (Fig. 6.3). Presenting ocular symptoms include photophobia, redness, pain, visual field defects, floaters, and diplopia [31]. The most common ophthalmic manifestation is chorioretinitis, often showing characteristic multifocal scattered or linear scars bilaterally [31]. Involvement of the macula can lead to central visual loss [31, 32]. Additional ocular features include anterior uveitis, retinal vasculitis, cotton wool spots, and pigmented and atrophic retinal scars [32]. Neuro-invasive disease can cause optic disc edema, ischemic optic neuritis, afferent pupillary defects, and cranial nerve six palsy [31]. Congenital transplacental transmission has been associated with congenital chorioretinal scarring [29–32].

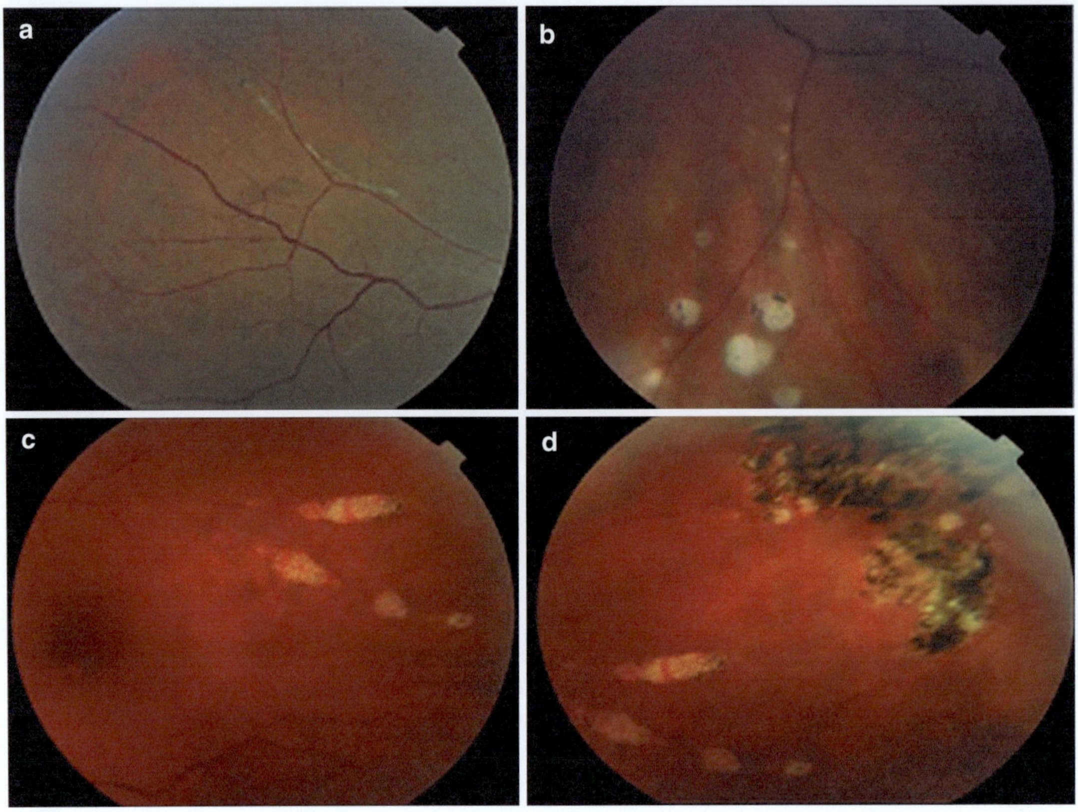

Fig. 6.3 Images showing retinopathy in four different patients with a history of West Nile virus [31]; https://doi.org/10.1371/journal.pone.0148898.g001 © Copyright Policy – open access; https://openi.nlm.nih.gov/

Chikungunya

The Chikungunya virus is a member of the genus *Alphavirus* and family *Togaviridae*. This virus reemerged from near extinction in India during an outbreak in 2005 and has continued to cause new infections ever since. This virus spreads though the bite of the infected *Aedes aegypti* and *Aedes albopictus* mosquito. There are four serotypes of Chikungunya virus: East-Central-South Africa, West Africa, Asian, and Indian Ocean lineages [33]. The word *chikungunya* is derived from the Nigerian Kimakonde word meaning "that which bends up" in reference to the stooped posture that patients may develop as a result of the arthritic symptoms of the disease.

The incubation period of Chikungunya ranges from 1 to 12 days. Symptoms include acute onset high-grade fever, headache, myalgias, and moderate-to-severe arthralgia that affects the extremities. More than 70% of people infected with Chikungunya are symptomatic [34]. The most common features of chikungunya infection are acute high-grade fever, crippling joint pain, and rash [35]. Headache, digestive illnesses, arthritis, fatigue, and conjunctivitis may occur as well [34, 35]. The disease is self-limiting, though a subset of patients will develop lifelong arthritis as a sequela. Severe cases can have life-threatening complications including meningitis, liver failure, and severe bleeding. The gold standard for diagnosing Chikungunya is by viral culture. As with other arboviruses, treatment is supportive, and there is no available vaccine for public use [35].

Ocular manifestations of chikungunya virus most commonly include iridocyclitis and retinitis, which have a generally benign clinical course [36]. Patients can present with redness, decreased or blurred vision, ocular pain, floaters, photophobia, diplopia, tearing, or irritation [36, 37]. Examination may show increased intraocular pressures. The anterior segment can show conjunctivitis, subconjunctival hemorrhage, episcleritis, corneal edema, keratitis, uveitis, and vitritis [36–38]. Retinal findings include macular edema, retinal whitening, and vasculitis. Chikungunya infection can also affect the optic nerve [36]. Neuroretinitis, optic dis edema, homonymous hemianopia, cranial nerve VI and VII palsies, and scotomas have been described [37]. Prognosis of ocular disease is good in those affected by chikungunya, with most patients achieving recovery of visual symptoms [38].

Virology and Diagnostic Testing for Arboviral Infections

Yellow Fever

The diagnosis of yellow fever may be established by demonstrating the presence of the virus or demonstration of an immune response to the presence of the virus. PCR of blood is the best for direct detection of the virus during infection. Virus isolation can be done by inoculation of mosquito or mammalian cell cultures, but the procedure is labor-intensive and time-consuming.

Serological testing for IgM antibodies against YFV provides indirect evidence of infection. Although a single sample provides a presumptive diagnosis, persistence of antibiotics from earlier vaccination can cause confusion. A rise in titer between acute and convalescent samples provides a more definitive serological diagnosis.

Dengue

Diagnostic tests for dengue include assays to detect the virus or its components (genome and antigen) or the host response to the virus, depending on the time of patient presentation. Viremia is detectable for roughly 4–5 days after the onset of fever and correlates closely with fever duration (RT-PCR). The virus may also be detected by testing for a virus-produced protein called NS1. There are commercially produced rapid diagnostic tests available to detect NS1 protein that require only 20 min to result, and the test does not require specialized laboratory techniques or equipment. Serological methods, such as enzyme-linked immunosorbent assays (ELISA), may confirm the presence of a recent or past infection, with the detection of IgM and IgG anti-dengue antibodies. IgM antibodies are detectable about 1 week after infection and are highest at 2–4 weeks after the onset of illness. They remain detectable for about 3 months. The presence of IgM is indicative of a recent DENV infection. IgG antibody levels take longer to develop than IgM, but IgG antibodies remain detectable for years. The presence of IgG is indicative of past infection [13].

Zika Virus

Zika virus infection is diagnosed by nucleic acid amplification testing (NAAT) on serum collected ≤7 days after symptom onset. Zika virus IgM antibody testing should be performed on NAAT-negative serum specimens or serum collected more than 7 days after the onset of symptoms. For symptomatic pregnant women, serum and urine specimens should be collected as soon as possible within 12 weeks of symptom onset for concurrent dengue and Zika virus NAATs and IgM antibody testing. Positive IgM antibody test results with negative NAAT results should be confirmed by neutralizing antibody tests when clinically or epidemiologically indicated, including for all pregnant women. Diagnostic guidelines are addressed at the US CDC website [39, 40].

West Nile Virus

Detection of IgM antibody in serum or cerebrospinal fluid (CSF) using the IgM antibody-capture enzyme-linked immunosorbent assay (MAC-ELISA) forms the cornerstone of West Nile virus diagnosis in most clinical settings. Because IgM antibody does not cross the blood-brain barrier, its presence in CSF indicates CNS infection [16]. The plaque-reduction neutralization test can help distinguish serologic cross-reactions among the flaviviruses, but the test is only available in reference laboratories. Nucleic acid amplification testing has utility in certain clinical settings as an adjunct to MAC-ELISA. Total leukocyte counts in peripheral blood typically are normal or slightly elevated. Examination of CSF of patients with neuroinvasive disease shows normal glucose. Virus detection is highly specific but is of limited value for routine diagnosis since viremia in humans is only found early in the course of disease (often before symptoms develop), is of low titer, and is short lived. Among patients with neuroinvasive disease, the sensitivity of nucleic acid testing using the PCR is less than 15 percent when testing serum or plasma and only about 55 percent for CSF [41].

Chikungunya

The diagnosis of Chikungunya infection is established by detection of chikungunya viral RNA via real-time reverse-transcription polymerase chain reaction (RT-PCR) or chikungunya virus serology. Laboratory diagnosis is generally made by testing serum or plasma to detect virus, viral nucleic acid, or virus-specific immunoglobulin IgM and neutralizing antibodies. Viral culture may detect virus in the first 3 days of illness; however, chikungunya virus should be handled under biosafety level (BSL) 3 conditions. During the first 8 days of illness, chikungunya viral RNA can often be identified in serum. Chikungunya virus antibodies normally develop toward the end of the first week of illness. Therefore, to definitively rule out the diagnosis, convalescent-phase samples should be obtained from patients whose acute-phase samples test negative [42].

Management

Dengue

There is no specific treatment for dengue fever. The best option to treat fever and myalgia is acetaminophen. NSAIDs (nonsteroidal anti-inflammatory drugs), such as ibuprofen and aspirin, should be avoided. These anti-inflammatory drugs inhibit platelet function, and in a disease with risk of hemorrhage, inhibition of platelet function may worsen the prognosis [43]. The first dengue vaccine, Dengvaxia® (CYD-TDV) developed by Sanofi Pasteur, was licensed in December 2015 and has now been approved by regulatory authorities in 20 countries. The vaccine is targeted for persons living in endemic areas, ranging from 9 to 45 years of age, who have had at least 1 documented dengue virus infection previously [44].

Yellow Fever

No specific antiviral treatment exists for yellow fever, though a cost-effective 17D yellow fever vaccine is available [9]. Supportive care is given to maximize tissue perfusion and reduce hemorrhagic complications [9].

Zika Virus

There is no specific treatment or preventive vaccine for Zika virus infection.

West Nile Virus

There is no specific treatment or preventive vaccine for WNV disease in humans.

Chikungunya

Treatment is symptomatic. There is currently no specific treatment or preventive vaccine for CHIKV infection in humans.

Management of Ocular Disease

There is no gold standard for treatment of arbovirus infections. Corticosteroid drops can be used to decrease inflammation and have shown to be useful in cases of Chikungunya virus [19, 30, 36]. Artificial tears and lubricating eye drops can provide relief from irritation and dryness. Pressure-lowering drops such as latanoprost and cycloplegics can be used to decrease intraocular pressures in select cases. Acyclovir, an antiviral medication, has been tried for treatment in a few cases [36, 45–47]. Cataract removal surgery may be indicated. Retinal disease may require surgeries including vitrectomy, retinal detachment repair, and laser ablation. However, necrosis and damage to the retinal cells are often not amenable to treatment [48].

Cases

Case 1 (Fig. 6.4)

A 33-year-old Central American female who developed a viral syndrome including headache, conjunctivitis, generalized rash, malaise and low-grade fever during an outbreak of Zika virus, dengue, and Chikungunya. Following resolution of her systemic symptoms, she developed vision loss to finger counting in both eyes.

Case 2 (Figs. 6.5 and 6.6)

A 13-year-old girl presented with painless loss of vision for the 2 weeks in the setting of fever, myalgias, headache, and chills. Visual acuity testing showed finger counting in the right eye and 3/200 in the left eye. Fundus examination revealed superficial retinal hemorrhages, Roth spots, and subhyaloid hemorrhages in both eyes.

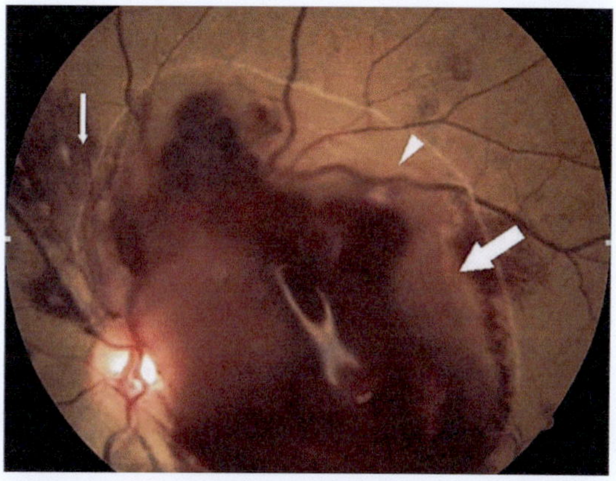

Fig. 6.5 Fundus photograph of the left eye showing Roth spots and subhyaloid hemorrhage. © Copyright Policy – open access. https://openi.nlm.nih.gov/

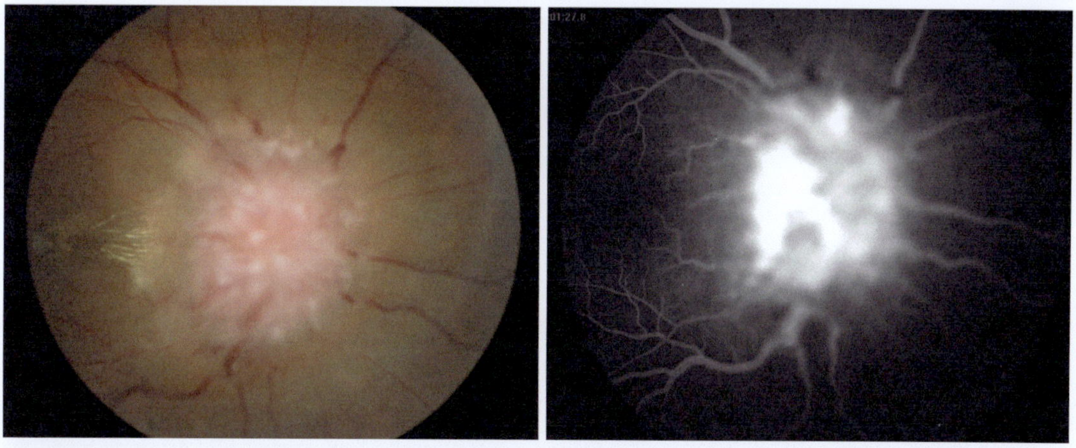

Fig. 6.4 Fundus photos showing severe optic disc edema with a macular star with exudates (left). A fluorescein angiogram showed intense leakage of the optic disc (right). Image courtesy of Dr. Steven Yeh, Atlanta, GA

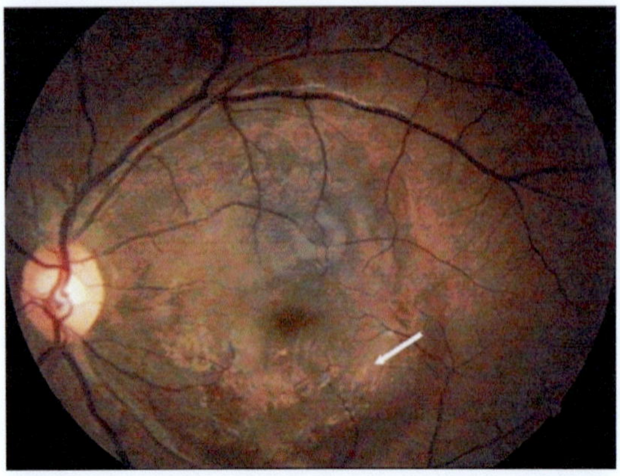

Fig. 6.6 Fundus photograph of the left eye 3 months after initial presentation, following treatment with laser hyaloidotomy. © Copyright Policy – open access. https://openi.nlm.nih.gov/

She was diagnosed with dengue hemorrhagic fever via enzyme-linked immunosorbent assay. The patient was treated with blood transfusions, and her eye manifestations were treated with laser hyaloidotomy. The vision in the treated eye improved from 3/200 to 20/30 and remained stable after 3 months.

Compliance with Ethical Requirements Sara L. Hojjatie, Lucileia Teixeira, Jessica G. Shantha, and John Johnson declare that they have no conflict of interest.

Steven Yeh declares that he has received consulting fees from Santen, Clearside Biomedical, and Bausch and Lomb.

References

1. Singh S, Farr D, Kumar A. Ocular manifestations of emerging flaviviruses and the blood-retinal barrier. Viruses. 2018;10:530. https://doi.org/10.3390/v10100530.
2. Bhatt S, Gething PW, Brady OJ, Messina JP, Farlow AW, Moyes CL, et al. The global distribution and burden of dengue. Nature. 2013;496:504–7. https://doi.org/10.1038/nature12060.
3. Patterson J, Sammon M, Garg M. Dengue, zika and chikungunya: emerging arboviruses in the new world. West J Emerg Med. 2016;17:671–9. https://doi.org/10.5811/westjem.2016.9.30904.
4. Rosenberg R, Ben BC. Vector-borne infections. Emerg Infect Dis. 2011;17:769–70. https://doi.org/10.3201/eid1705.110310.
5. Sharp TM, Fischer M, Muñoz-Jordán JL, Paz-Bailey G, Staples JE, Gregory CJ, et al. Dengue and zika virus diagnostic testing for patients with a clinically compatible illness and risk for infection with both viruses. MMWR Recomm Rep. 2019;68:1–10. https://doi.org/10.15585/mmwr.rr6801a1.
6. Roehrig JT, Nash D, Maldin B, Labowitz A, Martin DA, Lanciotti RS, et al. Persistence of virus-reactive serum immunoglobulin M antibody in confirmed west nile virus encephalitis cases. Emerg Infect Dis. 2003;9:376–9. https://doi.org/10.3201/eid0903.020531.
7. Paz-Bailey G, Rosenberg ES, Doyle K, Munoz-Jordan J, Santiago GA, Klein L, et al. Persistence of zika virus in body fluids -- final report. N Engl J Med. 2018;379:1234–43. https://doi.org/10.1056/NEJMoa1613108.
8. Munoz-Jordan JL. Diagnosis of zika virus infections: challenges and opportunities. J Infect Dis. 2017;216:S951–6. https://doi.org/10.1093/infdis/jix502.
9. Monath TP. Yellow fever: an update. Lancet Infect Dis. 2001;1:11–20. https://doi.org/10.1016/S1473-3099(01)00016-0.
10. Shantha JG, Yeh S, Acharya N. Insights from 2 outbreaks in southeastern Brazil: yellow fever retinopathy. JAMA Ophthalmol. 2019;137:1003. https://doi.org/10.1001/jamaophthalmol.2019.1936.
11. Vianello S, Silva de Souza G, Maia M, Belfort R, de Oliveira Dias JR. Ocular findings in yellow fever infection. JAMA Ophthalmol. 2019;137:300. https://doi.org/10.1001/jamaophthalmol.2018.6408.
12. Brandão-de-Resende C, Cunha LHM, Oliveira SL, Pereira LS, Oliveira JGF, Santos TA, et al. Characterization of retinopathy among patients with yellow fever during 2 outbreaks in Southeastern Brazil. JAMA Ophthalmol. 2019;137:996. https://doi.org/10.1001/jamaophthalmol.2019.1956.
13. Guzman MG, Harris E. Dengue. The Lancet. 2015;385:453–65. https://doi.org/10.1016/S0140-6736(14)60572-9.
14. Weaver SC, Vasilakis N. Molecular evolution of dengue viruses: Contributions of phylogenetics to understanding the history and epidemiology of the preeminent arboviral disease. Infect Genet Evol. 2009;9:523–40. https://doi.org/10.1016/j.meegid.2009.02.003.
15. Bacsal KE. Dengue-Associated Maculopathy. Arch Ophthalmol. 2007;125:501. https://doi.org/10.1001/archopht.125.4.501.
16. de Andrade GC, Ventura CV, Mello Filho PA, Maia M, Vianello S, Rodrigues EB. Arboviruses and the eye. Int J Retina Vitreous. 2017;3:4. https://doi.org/10.1186/s40942-016-0057-4.
17. Chia A. Electrophysiological findings in patients with dengue-related maculopathy. Arch Ophthalmol. 2006;124:1421. https://doi.org/10.1001/archopht.124.10.1421.
18. Li M, Zhang X, Ji Y, Ye B, Wen F. Acute macular neuroretinopathy in dengue fever: short-term

prospectively followed up case series. JAMA Ophthalmol. 2015;133:1329. https://doi.org/10.1001/jamaophthalmol.2015.2687.
19. Ng AW, Teoh SC. Dengue eye disease. Surv Ophthalmol. 2015;60:106–14. https://doi.org/10.1016/j.survophthal.2014.07.003.
20. Miner JJ, Diamond MS. Zika virus pathogenesis and tissue tropism. Cell Host Microbe. 2017;21:134–42. https://doi.org/10.1016/j.chom.2017.01.004.
21. Karimi O, Goorhuis A, Schinkel J, Codrington J, Vreden SGS, Vermaat JS, et al. Thrombocytopenia and subcutaneous bleedings in a patient with Zika virus infection. The Lancet. 2016;387:939–40. https://doi.org/10.1016/S0140-6736(16)00502-X.
22. de Paula FB, de Oliveira Dias JR, Prazeres J, Sacramento GA, Ko AI, Maia M, et al. Ocular Findings in Infants with Microcephaly Associated with Presumed Zika Virus Congenital Infection in Salvador. Brazil. JAMA Ophthalmol. 2016;134:529. https://doi.org/10.1001/jamaophthalmol.2016.0267.
23. Simonin Y, Erkilic N, Damodar K, Clé M, Desmetz C, Bolloré K, et al. Zika virus induces strong inflammatory responses and impairs homeostasis and function of the human retinal pigment epithelium. EBioMedicine. 2019;39:315–31. https://doi.org/10.1016/j.ebiom.2018.12.010.
24. Manangeeswaran M, Kielczewski JL, Sen HN, Xu BC, Ireland Derek DC, McWilliams IL, et al. ZIKA virus infection causes persistent chorioretinal lesions. Emerg Microbes Infect. 2018;7:1–15. https://doi.org/10.1038/s41426-018-0096-z.
25. Singh PK, Guest J-M, Kanwar M, Boss J, Gao N, Juzych MS, et al. Zika virus infects cells lining the blood-retinal barrier and causes chorioretinal atrophy in mouse eyes. JCI Insight. 2017:2. https://doi.org/10.1172/jci.insight.92340.
26. Zhu S, Luo H, Liu H, Ha Y, Mays ER, Lawrence RE, et al. p38MAPK plays a critical role in induction of a pro-inflammatory phenotype of retinal Müller cells following Zika virus infection. Antiviral Res. 2017;145:70–81. https://doi.org/10.1016/j.antiviral.2017.07.012.
27. Henry CR, Al-Attar L, Cruz-Chacón AM, Davis JL. Chorioretinal Lesions Presumed Secondary to Zika Virus Infection in an Immunocompromised Adult. JAMA Ophthalmol. 2017;135:386. https://doi.org/10.1001/jamaophthalmol.2017.0098.
28. Smithburn KC, Hughes TP, Burke AW, Paul JH. A Neurotropic Virus Isolated from the Blood of a Native of Uganda 1. Am J Trop Med Hyg. 1940;s1–20:471–92. https://doi.org/10.4269/ajtmh.1940.s1-20.471.
29. Priestley Y, Thiel M, Koevary SB. Systemic and ophthalmic manifestations of West Nile virus infection. Expert Rev. Ophthalmol. 2008;3:279–92. https://doi.org/10.1586/17469899.3.3.279.
30. Garg S, Jampol LM. Systemic and intraocular manifestations of West Nile virus infection. Surv Ophthalmol. 2005;50:3–13. https://doi.org/10.1016/j.survophthal.2004.10.001.
31. Hasbun R, Garcia MN, Kellaway J, Baker L, Salazar L, Woods SP, et al. West nile virus retinopathy and associations with long term neurological and neurocognitive sequelae. Plos One. 2016;11:e0148898. https://doi.org/10.1371/journal.pone.0148898.
32. Sivakumar RR, Prajna L, Arya LK, Muraly P, Shukla J, Saxena D, et al. Molecular diagnosis and ocular imaging of west nile virus retinitis and neuroretinitis. Ophthalmology. 2013;120:1820–6. https://doi.org/10.1016/j.ophtha.2013.02.006.
33. Thiberville SD, Moyen N, Dupuis-Maguiraga L, Nougairede A, Gould EA, et al. Chikungunya fever: Epidemiology, clinical syndrome, pathogenesis and therapy. Antiviral Res. 2013;99(3):345–70.
34. Thiberville SD, Moyen N, Dupuis-Maguiraga L, Nougairede A, Gould EA, Roques P, et al. Chikungunya fever: Epidemiology, clinical syndrome, pathogenesis and therapy. Antiviral Res. 2013; https://doi.org/10.1016/j.antiviral.2013.06.009.
35. Mohan A, Kiran DH, Manohar IC, Kumar DP. Epidemiology, clinical manifestations, and diagnosis of Chikungunya fever: lessons learned from the re-emerging epidemic. Indian J Dermatol. 2010;55(1):54–63. https://doi.org/10.4103/0019-5154.60355. PMID: 20418981; PMCID: PMC2856377
36. Mahendradas P, Ranganna SK, Shetty R, Balu R, Narayana KM, Babu RB, et al. Ocular manifestations associated with chikungunya. Ophthalmology. 2008;115(2):287–91. https://doi.org/10.1016/j.ophtha.2007.03.085. Epub 2007 Jul 12. PMID: 17631967
37. Mittal A, Mittal S, Bharati MJ, Ramakrishnan R, Saravanan S, Sathe PS. Optic neuritis associated with chikungunya virus infection in South India. Arch Ophthalmol. 2007;125(10):1381–6. https://doi.org/10.1001/archopht.125.10.1381. PMID: 17923547
38. Lalitha P, Rathinam S, Banushree K, Maheshkumar S, Vijayakumar R, Sathe P. Ocular involvement associated with an epidemic outbreak of chikungunya virus infection. Am J Ophthalmol. 2007;144(4):552–6. https://doi.org/10.1016/j.ajo.2007.06.002. Epub 2007 Aug 9. PMID: 17692276
39. Sharp TM, Fischer M, Muñoz-Jordán JL, Paz-Bailey G, Erin Staples J, Gregory CJ, et al. Dengue and zika virus diagnostic testing for patients with a clinically compatible illness and risk for infection with both viruses. MMWR Recomm Rep. 2019; https://doi.org/10.15585/MMWR.RR6801A1.
40. Dick GWA. Zika Virus (I). Isolations and serological specificity. Trans R Soc Trop Med Hyg. 1952; https://doi.org/10.1016/0035-9203(52)90042-4.
41. Nash D, Mostashari F, Fine A, Miller J, O'Leary D, Murray K, et al. The outbreak of West Nile virus infection in the New York City area in 1999. N Engl J Med. 2001; https://doi.org/10.1056/NEJM200106143442401.
42. Editors. Where can I order chikungunya virus testing? [Internet] Centers for Disease Control and Prevention;

2018 [cited 2020 April 10]. Available from: https://www.cdc.gov/chikungunya/hc/diagnostic.html
43. Waggoner JJ, Gresh L, Vargas MJ, Ballesteros G, Tellez Y, Soda KJ, et al. Viremia and Clinical Presentation in Nicaraguan Patients Infected with Zika Virus, Chikungunya Virus, and Dengue Virus. Clin Infect Dis. 2016;63(12):1584–90.
44. Editors. Dengue and severe dengue. [Internet] World Health Organization; 2020 [accessed cited 2020 April 4] Available from: https://www.who.int/news-room/fact-sheets/detail/dengue-and-severe-dengue
45. Murthy KR, Venkataraman N, Satish V, Babu K. Bilateral retinitis following chikungunya fever. Indian J Ophthalmol. 2008;56(4):329–31.
46. Murray KO, Baraniuk S, Resnick M, Arafat R, Kilborn C, Shallenberger R, et al. Clinical investigation of hospitalized human cases of West Nile virus infection in Houston, Texas, 2002–2004. Vector Borne Zoonotic Dis. 2008;8(2):167–74.
47. Larik A, Chiong Y, Lee LC, Ng YS. Longitudinally extensive transverse myelitis associated with dengue fever. BMJ Case Rep. 2012;2012 https://doi.org/10.1136/bcr.12.2011.5378.
48. Karesh JW, Mazzoli RA, Heintz SK. Ocular Manifestations of Mosquito-Transmitted Diseases. Mil Med. 2018; https://doi.org/10.1093/milmed/usx183.

Parasitic and Other Unusual Intraocular Infections

7

Matthew P. Nicholas, Sana Idrees, Angela P. Bessette, Jem Marie P. Golbin, and Jona M. Banzon

Abbreviations

AIDS	acquired immunodeficiency syndrome
CNV	choroidal neovascularization
CT	computed tomography
DSAEK	Descemet stripping automated endothelial keratoplasty
DUSN	diffuse unilateral subacute neuroretinitis
ELISA	enzyme-linked immunosorbent assay
ERG	electroretinogram
FA	fluorescein angiography
HIV	human immunodeficiency virus
IgM	immunoglobulin-M
IOL	intraocular lens
MCP	multifocal choroiditis and panuveitis
MRI	magnetic resonance imaging
Nd:YAG	neodymium-doped yttrium aluminum garnet
OCT	optical coherence tomography
OT	ocular toxocariasis
PCR	polymerase chain reaction
PIC	punctate inner choroidopathy
RB	retinoblastoma
RD	retinal detachment
RP	retinitis pigmentosa
RPE	retinal pigment epithelium
STD	sexually transmitted disease
TB	tuberculosis
TRD	tractional retinal detachment
UGH	uveitis-glaucoma-hyphema syndrome
VLM	visceral larva migrans

M. P. Nicholas
Eye Disease Consultants, West Hartford, CT, USA

S. Idrees
Monmouth Retina Consultants, Little Silver, NJ, USA
e-mail: sidrees@gwmail.gwu.edu

A. P. Bessette (✉)
Retina Associates of Western New York, Rochester, NY, USA
e-mail: abessette@retinawny.com

J. M. P. Golbin
University of the Philippines – College of Medicine, Quezon City, Philippines

J. M. Banzon
Department of Infectious Disease, Cleveland Clinic, Cleveland, OH, USA
e-mail: BANZONJ@ccf.org

Introduction

Intraocular Parasitic Infections

Protozoan Infections

Toxoplasmosis

Toxoplasma gondii is an intracellular protozoan parasite that is found worldwide. Serologic studies report an overall age-adjusted prevalence of

© Springer Nature Switzerland AG 2023
C. Y. Lowder et al. (eds.), *Emerging Ocular Infections*, Essentials in Ophthalmology,
https://doi.org/10.1007/978-3-031-24559-6_7

22.5% [1], with significant variations between regions. In some parts of the world, rates as high as 67% (France) [2] and 78% (Nigeria) [3] have been reported.

Members of the cat family are the definitive hosts for *Toxoplasma*. Cats shed large numbers of oocysts in feces, which become infective in the environment and can be consumed by a variety of intermediate hosts such as birds, rodents, and domesticated animals. Human infection can occur in a variety of ways. Infective oocysts can be ingested through contaminated food or water [4]. Consuming undercooked meat of intermediate hosts containing oocysts can also transmit toxoplasmosis. Blood transfusion and organ transplantation are also documented methods of transmission [5]. Lastly, transplacental infection can occur when the mother becomes infected with *Toxoplasma* during or immediately before pregnancy and can lead to congenital toxoplasmosis, which represents the first cases of ocular toxoplasmosis to be clearly described [6].

Pathogenesis Regardless of the route of initial systemic infection, primary intraocular invasion by *T. gondii* generally occurs via hematogenous spread, either as free tachyzoite or within mononuclear phagocytes. The mode of ocular entry is likely via the choroidal circulation with subsequent chorioretinal invasion [7, 8]. Invasion via the optic nerve from primary brain lesions has also been suggested. While cerebro-ocular spread may occur in some cases, it is not likely to be the typical route of ocular penetration. First, ocular toxoplasmosis may occur in the absence of toxoplasmosis encephalitis. Second, PCR analysis in murine models detected *T. gondii* in the retina and choroid several days earlier on average than in the optic nerve [9].

The majority of ocular toxoplasma infections are asymptomatic. However, ocular toxoplasmosis is a major cause of infectious posterior uveitis worldwide and was the second most common specific cause (after cytomegalovirus) of posterior uveitis in both academic and community general ophthalmology practices in one Los Angeles-based survey [10]. Numerous host and parasitic factors, which vary by geographic region, may affect virulence and both the systemic and localized ocular immune responses [7]. Initial symptomatic episodes of ocular toxoplasmosis typically occur around 30 years of age and generally represent reactivation of disease by release of tachyzoites previously encysted in chorioretinal scars. However, despite the classical teaching that initial infections are congenital, it appears that most infections actually occur in the postnatal period with a subclinical retinochoroiditis [11, 12]. Interestingly, older patients with primary infection may be at higher risk for clinical ocular toxoplasmosis, as multiple studies have shown that patients with ocular toxoplasmosis and serologic evidence of recently acquired infection are typically in their fifties [13]. Immunosuppression, especially concomitant HIV/AIDS, significantly increases the risk of severe ocular manifestations with either primary infection or reactivation.

Clinical Features The clinical presentation of ocular toxoplasmosis is variable [13–15]. Congenital toxoplasmosis may lead to devastating neurologic malformations and even fetal death, especially if acquired during early gestation. However, the most common presentation is a subclinical retinochoroiditis, which may be identified incidentally on exam years later as hyperpigmented chorioretinal scarring (often bilateral). Despite the small anatomical area occupied by the macula, toxoplasmic lesions have a predilection for the macula and posterior pole (Fig. 7.1a). While early infection is often subclinical, if untreated, a significant portion of affected children may develop severe vision loss within the first few years of life.

Active ocular toxoplasmosis in older children and adults typically presents with unilateral blurred vision and floaters. The classic finding is a "headlight-in-the-fog" appearance of a whitish, focal, necrotizing retinochoroiditis viewed through an overlying vitritis (see Fig. 7.1a). These lesions are often adjacent to old chorioretinal scars and are therefore referred to as "satellite lesions." Multifocal satellite lesions of different chronicity and/or focal retinochoroiditis in the absence of prior scars should raise suspicion for

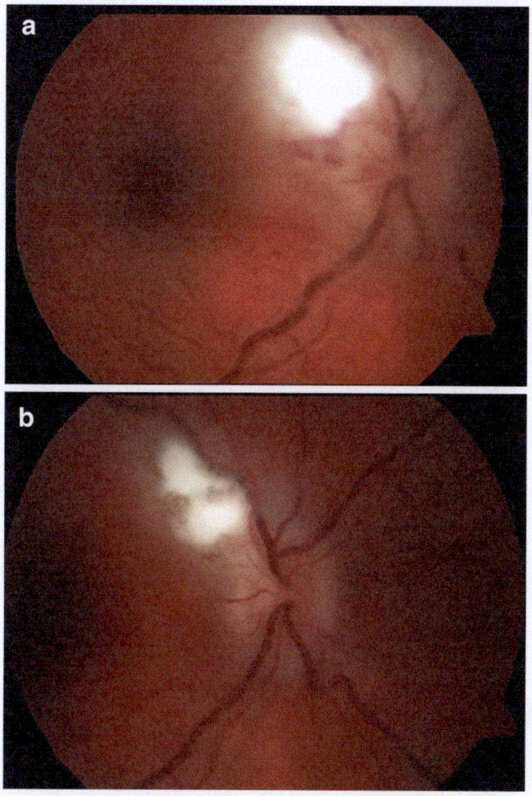

Fig. 7.1 (**a**) Fundus photograph demonstrating a classic "headlight-in-the-fog" appearance of a focal whitish retinochoroiditis with overlying vitritis, as well as optic nerve edema. (**b**) Appearance after 9 days of treatment, showing decreased vitritis and optic nerve edema, as well as consolidation of the chorioretinal lesion. Images courtesy of Careen Lowder

an alternative diagnosis (e.g., tuberculosis, syphilis, toxocariasis, viral acute retinal necrosis, or lymphoma) or an immunocompromised host (elderly patients, those on steroids or chemotherapy, those infected with HIV, etc.). Vitritis may be mild or absent in immunocompromised patients.

Despite the aforementioned classic presentation, a number of other findings and complications may occur [15], some of which may precede retinochoroiditis. Patients may complain of pain or photophobia resulting from a "spill-over" anterior uveitis; more rarely, the anterior chamber reaction may be granulomatous. This may lead to uveitic glaucoma. Perivascular lesions may cause retinal vasculitis (typically a phlebitis with venous sheathing, and less commonly a segmental arteritis), which can result in branch retinal vascular occlusions. As with other forms of posterior uveitis, optic disc edema and macular edema are relatively common. Vitreous bands may form in chronic cases. Rarer presentations include a *Bartonella*-like neuroretinitis with or without macular star, a retinitis pigmentosa-like pigmentary retinopathy, and punctate outer retinal toxoplasmosis (PORT), typically seen in immunocompromised patients and characterized by multifocal clusters of deep retinal lesions with associated subretinal fluid and minimal vitritis.

In immunocompetent hosts, retinochoroiditis is typically self-limited and resolves within 6 to 8 weeks, leaving a sharply demarcated, hyperpigmented chorioretinal scar. Recurrences are common, even after treatment that successfully terminates the initial episode. Potential chronic complications leading to permanent vision loss include cataract, retinal detachment (RD), macular edema, macular scar, epiretinal membrane, optic atrophy, and choroidal neovascularization.

Laboratory Testing Ocular toxoplasmosis is typically a clinical diagnosis based on fundoscopic findings. In equivocal cases or if the exam is limited by vitritis, PCR and antibody testing of intraocular fluid may be useful. While PCR is not highly sensitive, it is highly specific. When assessing intraocular IgG levels, determining the ratio of the relative abundance of *T. gondii*-specific IgG in intraocular fluid versus plasma, also known as the Goldmann-Witmer ratio, provides a sensitive indicator of local intraocular immune response. A ratio of greater than 3 indicates elevated local antibody production. Combining multiple diagnostic modalities may yield improved overall sensitivity [16, 17]. Optical coherence tomography (OCT) can localize chorioretinal lesions as well as identify and quantify macular and optic disc edema. B-scan ultrasound is useful in identifying RD in the setting of hazy media with poor fundoscopic views.

Management Encysted, dormant parasites in old chorioretinal scars do not require antiparasitic treatment. Active ocular toxoplasmosis typically resolves spontaneously in about 6–8 weeks.

Therefore, close observation is reasonable in cases with single, fairly peripheral lesions, good vision, and mild symptoms. Treatment is indicated in all cases of immunocompromised patients, newly infected pregnant women, and neonates with congenital infections (typically for the entire first year of life regardless of retinal findings). In other cases, relative indications for treatment include sight-threatening lesions involving the fovea, optic nerve head, papillomacular bundle, or major vessels; severe vitritis; multiple active lesions; or chronic course.

The effectiveness of antimicrobial treatment remains controversial; some nonrandomized studies show a reduction in lesion size and frequency of recurrence, but other benefits such as reduction in disease duration could not be demonstrated. The "classic" antimicrobial regimen consists of the combination of oral sulfadiazine, pyrimethamine, leucovorin, and corticosteroids for 4 to 6 weeks [18]. An alternative regimen is trimethoprim/sulfamethoxazole (80 mg/400 mg) twice daily with prednisone, which was shown to have similar efficacy in one prospective randomized trial [19]. Other alternatives include clindamycin, atovaquone, spiramycin, and azithromycin alone or in combination [20].

Intravitreal clindamycin in combination with intravitreal dexamethasone may be an effective alternative to the aforementioned systemic therapies, but patients with newly acquired systemic infection (i.e., positive IgM serology) or who are immunocompromised should receive systemic therapy [21]. Intravitreal clindamycin may be preferable in pregnant women to avoid systemic exposure.

Anterior uveitis, if present, is treated with topical steroid drops, cycloplegics, and ocular hypotensives if indicated. Unlike intravitreal dexamethasone, intraocular triamcinolone is contraindicated in cases of toxoplasmosis due to the potential for a fulminant, catastrophic panuveitis. Systemic steroids are typically started within 48 hours of antiparasitic therapy, only in immunocompetent patients and never in the absence of antibiotics. Steroids should be deferred if there is any question about alternative diagnoses such as syphilis or TB. Diagnostic and therapeutic vitrectomy may be useful when the diagnosis is uncertain or in cases of dense, nonclearing vitritis or other complications, such as RD, that require surgical intervention.

Nematode Infections

Toxocariasis

Toxocara species are roundworms that infect a variety of wild and domestic definitive hosts. They have complex life cycles that can involve one or multiple hosts. Highest prevalence of infection is observed in developing countries and within lower socioeconomic strata, although the disease is found globally [22]. Definitive hosts, such as dogs and cats, shed eggs in feces which then become infectious in the environment. These can be ingested by paratenic hosts, where they hatch into larvae in the digestive tract. Larvae penetrate the gut wall, migrating into various tissues where they encyst. Humans can become infected by ingesting infective eggs in contaminated food, water, or soil. Encysted larvae in undercooked meat or viscera of infected paratenic hosts can also be consumed by humans. Larvae are released in the human small intestine, penetrate the wall, and migrate to various organs including lungs, liver, muscle, and brain [23].

Pathogenesis After penetration of the intestinal wall, larvae disseminate via hematogenous and lymphatic routes. They are capable of entering numerous tissues (visceral larva migrans, VLM) including the eyes (ocular toxocariasis, OT), most likely via the choroidal circulation. Ultimately, the worm dies and is encapsulated in an eosinophilic granuloma [24]. While VLM tends to affect children younger than 3 years old, OT occurs more often in older children or young adults, is generally present in the absence of concurrent VLM, and is associated with a lower parasitic load. It is almost always unilateral. Inflammation is thought to occur due to antigens released from dead larvae.

Clinical Features There are multiple characteristic presentations of OT, including (1) chronic endophthalmitis, (2) localized macular/peripapillary granuloma, and (3) peripheral retinal granuloma. Depending on the chronicity, extensive chorioretinal scarring may be present. *Toxocara* infection is also associated with diffuse unilateral subacute neuroretinitis (DUSN).

The average age at presentation is about 12 years old, and the typical complaint is unilateral decreased vision. Patients may have pain, photophobia, and floaters. Although anterior uveitis is possible in severe cases, the anterior segment is generally quiet. Leukocoria may result from posterior inflammation or retinal granulomas, the appearance of which can be difficult to distinguish from retinoblastoma (RB). Features more characteristic of RB include lack of inflammation, presence of retinal calcifications, rapid lesion growth, and younger age at presentation.

Chronic endophthalmitis is more typical in younger patients and is associated with the worst vision at presentation. Vitritis and chorioretinitis are typical and leukocoria and strabismus are common. A retinal granuloma may be present but obscured by the vitritis. Potential complications include cystoid macular edema, exudative RD, formation of vitreous cyclitic membranes, and vitreoretinal traction bands with resultant tractional RD (TRD). Less commonly, a dense, peripheral exudate similar to snowbanking may occur.

The location of retinal granulomas significantly influences clinical manifestations. Macular and peripapillary granulomas appear as yellow-white, elevated lesions, which are typically 1 to 2 disc diameters in size. Although foveal involvement can lead to severe vision loss, acuity is generally fairly well preserved as these lesions are often seen in the absence of vitritis and have a relatively low propensity for formation of vitreoretinal traction bands. Peripheral granulomas have a similar appearance, but are more often associated with vitreoretinal traction, leading to dragging of the vessels and retina similar in appearance to retinopathy of prematurity and familial exudative vitreoretinopathy. These can cause TRD. As a result, peripheral granulomas are generally associated with worse vision loss than those at the posterior pole.

Laboratory Testing The diagnosis of OT is predominantly clinical. ELISA serologic testing has a high sensitivity and specificity but may be negative in a significant number of cases. In addition, *Toxocara* seroprevalence in the general population is fairly high, making positive results of very limited value outside the appropriate clinical scenario. Vitreous biopsy with calculation of the Goldmann-Witmer ratio may be more useful than serologic testing alone. Histopathology of a vitreous biopsy may also demonstrate organisms directly. PCR has been attempted but has not been successful even in documented cases of OT [25]. Unlike VLM, the level of eosinophilia does not necessarily correlate with the severity of parasite burden in OT.

B-scan ultrasound is useful for assessing for vitreous membranes, masses, and RDs when the fundoscopic view is obscured. B-scan can also be used to assess for retinal calcium deposits, which are characteristic of retinoblastoma, but not of OT. Computed tomography (CT) can also detect calcium deposits, but should be used judiciously in cases of possible retinoblastoma, especially if there is a family history of RB, due to the carcinogenicity of ionizing radiation [26]. MRI has poor sensitivity for detecting calcium.

Management The mainstays of treatment are local and/or systemic corticosteroids. Because the inflammation is thought to be due to antigens released by dead organisms, antihelminthic drugs are not used routinely. If antihelminthic drugs are employed, they should always be co-administered with steroids. Vitrectomy for lysis of vitreoretinal adhesions may be useful in cases of sight-threatening retinal distortion or TRD. In rare cases in which larvae are identified on clinical examination, laser photocoagulation can be considered.

Diffuse Unilateral Subacute Neuroretinitis (DUSN)

Pathogenesis DUSN is caused by a subretinal, motile nematode and typically occurs in young, otherwise healthy individuals, often in their early teenage years. The causative organism has never been definitively isolated. One case of physical removal of the worm by vitrectomy with retinectomy and aspiration has been reported, but histopathology was not possible due to specimen deterioration [27]. Worms of two distinct sizes have been observed, and *Toxocara canis* and *Ancylostoma caninum* (both approximately 400 μm–1 mm in length) as well as *Baylisascaris procyonis* (1.5–2 mm in length) have been implicated [24]. The pathogenesis appears to involve local toxic effects of nematode byproducts left in the subretinal space as the organism migrates, and the associated inflammatory response is variable [28].

Clinical Features As its name implies, DUSN is characterized by the insidious onset of monocular neuroretinitis with associated vision loss. Early on, the severity of vision loss is often out of proportion to the clinical examination. If untreated, patients can suffer profound vision loss due to diffuse retinal damage. During these stages, patients may experience loss of color vision and nyctalopia. Despite its name, there have been reports of bilateral DUSN [29].

Early stages of infection are characterized by recurrent, evanescent clusters of gray-white or yellow-white outer retinal and choroidal lesions, which fade over a period of days and are often associated with vitritis and optic nerve edema. Some cases are associated with perivasculitis resembling retinal sarcoidosis [28]. On careful exam, a nematode may be seen migrating in the subretinal space, usually near the inflammatory lesions, but this represents the minority of cases. Gass et al. found subretinal worms in only 2 of 36 cases in the original case series which identified nematodes as the probable cause [30]. In the absence of this pathognomonic finding, the differential diagnosis is broad and includes numerous causes of posterior uveitis and panuveitis, such as sarcoidosis, multiple evanescent white dot syndrome, OT, and other causes of neuroretinitis.

Intermediate stages are characterized by multifocal chorioretinal scars that may resemble ocular histoplasmosis, multifocal choroiditis and panuveitis (MCP), and punctate inner choroidopathy (PIC). After months to years of chronic infection, progressive vision loss and retinal destruction occur. This ultimately yields an appearance similar to end-stage retinitis pigmentosa (RP), with RPE degeneration and chorioretinal scarring, optic atrophy, and arteriolar narrowing. For this reason, DUSN is sometimes referred to as "unilateral retinal wipeout syndrome" [31]. Late CNV may develop in some cases [30].

Laboratory Testing DUSN is a clinical diagnosis and systemic testing is generally unhelpful. Fundus photography can be useful in locating the nematode. ERG is subnormal even in the early stages, but, in contrast to tapetoretinal degenerations, is not completely extinguished [24]. OCT and fluorescein angiography (FA) may be useful in assessing the extent of retinal and vascular damage. In early disease, chorioretinal lesions block early and stain late on FA, and there may be perivascular leakage [28]. OCT may demonstrate disruption of the photoreceptor layer within weeks of symptom onset [28]. OCT has also been used to directly demonstrate subretinal nematodes [32].

Management Steroids alone achieve only transient improvement in inflammation, but can be useful as a temporizing measure early in the disease. They may also be useful in reducing vitritis and thereby improving the fundoscopic view for both diagnosis and treatment [33]. The definitive treatment is killing the causative organism, either by antihelminthic pharmacotherapy or direct laser photocoagulation of the subretinal nematode. After killing the worm, vision generally stabilizes and may even improve. However, there have been cases of relentless progression even after apparently successful laser therapy [32].

The preferred treatment is direct laser photocoagulation. Identification of the worm may require prolonged serial examinations, but typically is unsuccessful. Larger worms may not be instantly killed after a single laser shot and may subsequently retreat, so it is important to begin laser application when the worm is a safe distance from the fovea. Worms usually exhibit negative phototaxis (migration away from light), which can be utilized to direct them outside the macula before photocoagulation. After immobilization and presumed killing, barrier/grid laser can be applied around the organism. It is prudent to obtain post-treatment photos for later comparison as there have been cases of worms surviving, migrating, and requiring repeat photocoagulation [28, 34]. Photocoagulation has not been associated with a marked exacerbation of inflammation, which is presumably due to destruction and denaturing of nematode antigens.

In the majority of cases in which no organism is seen, laser photocoagulation may still be considered over recently developed lesions, based on the presumption that the nematode is present but simply obscured by the retinal whitening [35]. This approach may also be employed in conjunction with pharmacotherapy, as described below.

Antihelminthic treatment with thiabendazole or albendazole, which has a better side effect profile, is appropriate when no organism can be identified directly. Treatment may also immobilize the nematode and thereby increase the chances of identification and diagnosis. It can also be used as an adjunctive therapy to photocoagulation and may eliminate systemic infection that could lead to ocular reinvasion even after successful laser treatment. Antihelminthics are thought to be of limited efficacy in some cases due to sequestration of the nematode behind the blood-retinal barrier. For this reason, antihelmenthics may be more effective in the presence of vitritis [36]. Perivascular focal or grid laser may also be effective as a means of breaching the blood-retinal barrier and allowing penetration of antihelminthic drugs to the subretinal space [28, 35]. Successful treatment is often heralded 7–10 days after administration by a focal area of acute retinitis (due to the death of the worm) and simultaneous resolution of the other areas of inflammation [28].

Loiasis

Life Cycle/Mode of Transmission Considered a filarial nematode, the *Loa loa* parasite is transmitted to humans via the bite of the tabanid fly, genus *Chrysops*. *Loa loa* parasites begin their life as microfilariae that can be ingested by a day-biting *Chrysops* fly from a previously infected human. Within the fly, the parasite begins to grow eventually maturing into its infective form, the third-stage filarial larvae. These infectious larvae enter a human host during the fly's next meal [37]. Upon entering the human host, the larvae quickly invade the dermis and subcutaneous tissues where they can travel throughout the body via the lymphatics [38]. The filariae reside in these tissues where they further mature until reaching adulthood. Subsequently, the adult worms then reproduce, with the female worms releasing thousands of sheathed microfilariae into the host's lymphatics and then to the bloodstream. The majority of the microfilariae remain in the pulmonary circulation, which serves as a reservoir. At this stage, the microfilariae can now be found in the host's blood (to be ingested by another *Chrysops* fly) and, rarely, in other bodily fluids such as urine, saliva, and cerebrospinal fluid [39].

Epidemiological/Geographical Distribution Loiasis is native to the continent of Africa, particularly in West and Central Africa, encompassing countries such as Benin, Sudan, and Uganda [40].

Diagnostics Diagnosis of loiasis is confirmed by visualization of the microfilariae within the blood or other body tissues. However, the periodicity of the parasite lowers the sensitivity of this method [40]; hence, serological assays were developed. The ELISA test for *Loa loa* antigen has a high sensitivity but low specificity due to cross-reactivity with other parasitic infections such as *Strongyloides stercoralis*. The most specific and sensitive diagnostic is PCR detection [41].

Systemic Manifestations Loiasis has a latency period of several months to years [42]. There are two highly specific signs of loiasis—the first is the visualization of the worm under the conjunctiva of the eye. The second most specific sign is known as "Calabar swelling" which presents as a non-pitting, non-tender edema of the limbs, usually the forearms. The Calabar swelling spontaneously resolves but may recur on different sites of the body [43].

Other manifestations include arthralgia, a papular pruritic rash, usually on the arms, hematuria, or proteinuria—sometimes ranging into nephrotic syndrome, neurologic symptoms such as headache, sensory disturbance, and cranial nerve deficits [44–47].

Ocular Manifestations Both adult worms and microfilariae of *Loa loa* may affect the eye. The most common location of invasion is subconjunctival, but observation of thread-like, adult *Loa loa* worms in the anterior chamber has been reported numerous times [48–54]. In these cases, it is unclear whether the adult worm penetrates the sclera as it migrates, or whether the larva first invades the eye and then matures. Anterior chamber infestation can be associated with severe anterior uveitis (with or without hypopyon), cataract, and corneal edema. Treatment is generally surgical removal, anterior chamber washout, and systemic antihelminthic treatment.

Onchocerciasis (River Blindness)

Life Cycle/Mode of Transmission Human infection by the microfilaria *Onchocerca volvulus* occurs when an infected *Simulium* blackfly bites a human host. The infective stage of the parasite is the third stage microfilariae that can transfer from the vector and enter the human body through the bite. From the site of entry, the parasite then burrows into the subcutaneous tissues where they mature into adulthood. The interplay between the human body and the parasite results in the formation of nodules around the parasite [55]. *O. volvulus* has the ability to modulate the immune response of its host, resulting in significant immunosuppression with higher parasite burden [56]. The adult worms reproduce within the subcutaneous tissue and release microfilariae. These microfilariae can then travel throughout the body via the subcutaneous tissues or through the lymphatics. A small percentage of the microfilariae can enter the peripheral blood from where they can be ingested by the *Simulium* fly again and continue their development [57].

Geographical Distribution/Epidemiology Onchocerciasis is a disease mostly seen in sub-Saharan Africa. However, it is also rarely found in other tropical regions such as South America, particularly in Brazil and Venezuela [57]. The *Simulium* fly is known to live near running water, placing agricultural workers near rivers and streams at an increased risk [57].

Systemic Manifestations Infection with *O. volvulus* usually manifests with dermatologic and ophthalmologic features. Parasite movement and the host inflammatory response can cause an eruption of pruritic rashes during the migration of the microfilariae, appearance of depigmented skin patches, and loss of skin elasticity [55, 58].

Ocular Manifestations Ocular manifestations of onchocerciasis result from invasion of ocular tissues by *Onchocerca volvulus* microfilariae after initial dermal infection. The exact mechanism of ocular invasion is not known [59], but it has been shown that microfilariae migrate from the conjunctiva into the cornea [60, 61]. Ocular invasion may also occur via the bloodstream or along the nerves [14], Both dermal and ocular manifestations are thought to result from inflammation, particularly a Th_2 response, following death of the parasite (either due to natural attrition or chemotherapy), rather than from direct histologic injury by the parasite [59]. This may be due to release of *Wolbachia* bacteria, which are known to endosymbiotically infect the microfilariae [14, 62]. There is evidence that a significant feature of the host immune response (e.g., blocking antibodies and inhibitory cytokines) is in fact aimed at limiting local inflammation [63].

Clinical Features *O. volvulus* strains endemic to savannah regions appear to be more oculoinvasive and also more oculopathogenic compared to strains endemic to the rainforests [64]. Onchocerciasis can affect virtually any ocular tissue, leading to conjunctivitis and chemosis; punctate keratitis (subepithelial "snowflake opacities"); sclerosing keratitis and ultimately blindness via complete corneal opacification; intraocular worm with anterior uveitis; secondary glaucoma; papillitis; and chronic chorioretinitis with diffuse retinal atrophy [14]. Live microfilariae may be seen by slit lamp migrating in the cornea or suspended in the anterior chamber or vitreous, and visualization may be aided by prone positioning immediately before examination [65].

Laboratory Testing In addition to serology and histopathologic analysis (traditionally, skin-snip biopsy or sclerocorneal punch biopsy), testing is also available for urine and tear fluid by dip-stick antigen detection [66, 67] and PCR [65, 68].

Management Systemic treatment with antihelminthics (ivermectin, moxidectin, suramin) is combined with doxycycline, which kills symbiotic *Wolbachia* and thereby inhibits microfilarial embryogenesis. Systemic or topical steroids and cycloplegics are used to manage ocular inflammation. Surgical intervention may be indicated to address specific associated complications, such as corneal opacity, cataract, and glaucoma.

Cestode Infections

Cysticercosis

Life Cycle/Mode of Transmission Cysticercosis arises from infection with the larval stage of the pork tapeworm, *Taenia solium*, following the ingestion of *T. solium* eggs [69]. This cycle is usually related to close contact with a tapeworm carrier and consumption of food or water contaminated by *T. solium* eggs, rather than infected pork. Human cysticercosis is found worldwide, although the prevalence is higher in areas of poor sanitation, particularly in rural areas of developing countries where pigs and humans live side by side [70].

Pathogenesis Ingested *T. solium* eggs hatch in the intestine, and the larvae penetrate the intestinal wall. The larvae can spread hematogenously to any structure of the eye or orbit. They most frequently enter the eye via choroidal circulation after passing through the short posterior ciliary arteries. However, optic nerve head involvement has been reported and would suggest entry via the central retinal artery [71]. The larvae generally invade the subretinal space at the posterior pole. From there, they migrate and in some cases penetrate the retina to enter the vitreous cavity. Rarely, they may invade anterior chamber via the angle or ciliary body circulation or via transpupillary migration from the vitreous in aphakic patients [72]. After ocular invasion, the larvae encyst, forming a structure referred to as the cysticercus. As the larvae die, the cysticerci leak antigens and toxins into the surrounding tissues, which leads to intense local inflammation. Over time, the dead cysts eventually calcify [72].

Clinical Features Patients are generally young and otherwise healthy. Presentation is variable and may affect any part of the eye and its adnexae [72]. Intraocular manifestations depend primarily on whether the larvae remain subretinal or invade the vitreous. Patients may complain of eye pain, photophobia, floaters, and vision loss. There may be leukocoria, depending on the location of the parasite. However, asymptomatic infection is also possible. Observation of a motile cysticercus is pathognomonic. This appears as a whitish, translucent vesicle (typically spherical but sometimes multilobular) measuring a few millimeters in diameter. The cyst has an eccentric, dense, white opacity (receptaculum capitis) corresponding to an invagination in the cyst wall that contains the developing scolex (head) of the tapeworm. In some cases, the scolex may be exvaginated. The scolex often undulates in response to photostimulation.

Cysticerci may be observed in the conjunctiva, vitreous, subretinal space, or rarely anterior chamber. Vitritis is more frequent than anterior uveitis, which may be granulomatous [73], especially in the early stages of infection. Vitritis can lead to formation of vitreous bands and retinal traction. Subretinal involvement may cause chorioretinitis, epiretinal membrane, macular hole, exudative RD, proliferative vitreoretinopathy, retinal neovascularization, and vasculitis [72, 73]. Other potential complications include cataract, uveitic glaucoma [74], pupillary block glaucoma due to posterior synechiae or direct pupillary obstruction by the cysticercus [75], and neovascular glaucoma [76]. Vision loss can be severe, and prolonged infection may result in phthisis bulbi. While observation of a cysticercus is pathognomonic, the differential in uncertain cases includes other causes of leukocoria, choroidal tumors, and exudative RD, as well as other parasitic infections, such as toxoplasmosis, toxocariasis, and DUSN.

New seizures in the setting of ocular or other systemic findings of cysticercosis should raise suspicion for neurocysticercosis. In some cases, extraparenchymal subarachnoid involvement is associated with an elongated, racemose configuration of the parasite, though similar lesions may be observed in other cestode infections as well. For example, a case of disseminated *Versteria* with a subretinal cyst diagnosed through direct molecular analysis was recently reported [77].

Laboratory Testing The diagnosis is predominantly clinical. Eosinophilia and ELISA serologic testing from peripheral blood are poorly sensitive for ocular infection, but may have greater utility with anterior chamber paracentesis. Histopathology can confirm the diagnosis after surgical removal. In equivocal cases, PCR analysis of surgical specimens may be useful [77].

Ultrasonography may be used to assess for RD as well as to demonstrate the cysticercus, which appears as a thin-walled, internally hypoechoic mass with a hyperechoic scolex suspended from the inner wall ("hanging drop" sign) [78]. CT may also demonstrate cysticerci, especially after calcification. CT and MRI help with assessing cerebral involvement. OCT can identify subretinal cysts [79].

Management Surgical removal of all intraocular cysticerci with pre- and postoperative systemic steroids is the treatment of choice. Although antihelminthics such as praziquantel and albendazole may be necessary to treat systemic or cerebral manifestations, antihelminthics carry a substantial risk of inducing panuveitis secondary to larval death. Systemic therapy should therefore be avoided in isolated ocular cysticercosis. Multiple surgical techniques have been utilized to remove the parasite, including retinotomy and sclerotomy to access the subretinal space. While early literature advocated removing the cysts in toto to avoid intraocular release of parasitic antigens, pars plana vitrectomy with in vivo cyst lysis (i.e., removal by intraocular disruption and aspiration with the vitrector) has been shown to be safe and effective likely owing to the copious intraocular irrigation inherent to modern vitrectomy [80].

For anterior chamber involvement, viscoexpression [81–83] is a safe and effective method of removing even large cysts in toto without the risk of direct manipulation with instruments. The anterior chamber is filled with viscoelastic through a keratome incision, the posterior lip of which is then depressed, leading to egress of both the viscoelastic and the cysticercus. In some cases, simultaneous injection of additional viscoelastic via a separate paracentesis and use of a glide instrument via the main incision may help direct viscoelastic flow, maintain the anterior chamber, and prevent accidental displacement of the cyst posteriorly [83]. Regardless of the technique employed, care should be taken to ensure all cysts have been removed, especially prior to administering systemic antihelminthics.

Echinococcosis

Life Cycle/Mode of Transmission The *Echinococcus granulosus* tapeworm makes its way into the human body through accidental ingestion of tapeworm eggs [84]. The tapeworm begins its life cycle as eggs released within the small intestine of the carnivorous definitive hosts, such as foxes, dogs, or lions [85]. Upon defecation, the eggs are released into the environment from where they can contaminate vegetation and be ingested by an intermediate host such as sheep or other livestock. Within the intermediate host, the eggs mature into hydatid cysts and infect the definitive hosts upon consumption of their meat [86].

Humans may ingest the eggs through improperly washed produce or through interactions with animals that have picked up the eggs on their fur [87, 88]. Once inside the body, the eggs will mature into cysts after roughly 5 days [89].

Within the human body, *E. granulosus* cysts are most frequently seen in the liver followed by the lungs, kidneys, and spleen [90].

Geographical Distribution and Epidemiology *E. granulosus*, the species implicated in causing cystic echinococcosis, is found globally. *E. multilocularis*, which causes alveolar echinococcosis, is usually seen in North America and in northern and central Eurasia. *E. vogeli* and *E. oligarthrus*, which cause the more infrequent polycystic echinococcosis, are endemic to Central and South America [84, 91].

Diagnostics Identification of the cysts is key in making the diagnosis. This can be done through various imaging modalities such as ultrasonography, CT scan, and X-rays. Antibodies in blood may be detected in some cases. Aspiration and analysis of the cyst fluid via ELISA are a highly sensitive test; however, there is noted cross-reactivity with other cestode infections [90].

Systemic Manifestations Three clinical diseases result from *Echinococcus* infections: cystic echinococcosis, alveolar echinococcosis, and polycystic echinococcosis. The manifestations of the different syndromes result from the mass effect of the cysts. Liver cysts can cause abdominal pain, hepatomegaly, cholestasis, and portal hypertension, among others. Lung cysts can cause cough, dyspnea, and pleuritis, among others. Brain cysts can cause neurologic deficits depending on their location within the brain. Complications such as cyst rupture or secondary infection may occur. The contents of the cyst are highly immunogenic and can result in anaphylaxis. New metastatic cysts can also form after rupture of the original cysts causing secondary cystic echinococcosis [84, 90].

Ocular Manifestations Intraocular involvement is rare, but may present as a choroidal mass [92] or an intraocular cyst [75, 93]. While treatment of orbital cysts is surgical with concomitant antihelminthic and steroid therapy [14], the aforementioned cases of intraocular involvement were associated with either death of the patient or complete loss of the eye requiring enucleation.

Ectoparasites: Arthropods

Ophthalmomyiasis Interna

Pathogenesis Ophthalmomyiasis interna refers to intraocular invasion by larvae of any species of oestrid flies (botflies). In animal hosts, after deposition of eggs on the skin by adult flies, the larvae hatch, penetrate the skin, and migrate to the dorsal region, where they mature over a period of months [94]. Although the parasite does not appear to complete its life cycle in humans, ocular and adnexal ophthalmomyiasis are both known to occur, presumably due to aberrant larval migration aided by the secretion of proteolytic enzymes [14]. It is not known if oviposition on humans occurs naturally or if cases arise instead from exposure to infested animals or animal pelts.

Myiasis is associated with poor hygiene and low socioeconomic status [95]. Living in proximity to cattle also increases the risk of infestation [96]. Open wounds tend to attract the flies which is an additional risk factor for infestation [97].

Clinical Features Larvae may invade any structure of the globe, including the anterior chamber, vitreous, and subretinal spaces, with associated inflammatory reaction. In the subretinal space, the larvae may leave gray-white tracks in the RPE as they migrate [14]. Potential complications include chorioretinitis, vitritis, iridocyclitis, fibrovascular proliferation, focal hemorrhages, focal exudative detachment, lens dislocation, total RD, and loss of the eye. The diagnosis is made principally by the direct observation of a 1- to 2-mm translucent worm or maggot within the eye.

Laboratory Testing Diagnosis is mainly clinical, though definitive identification of the responsible species may be aided by light microscopy/histopathology, Western blot analysis, and electron microscopy of an isolated specimen. Electron microscopy may be employed even on small larval fragments, as they may contain characteristic features of external morphology that allow species identification [98].

Management Treatment is generally intraocular or systemic steroid administration with either vitrectomy, which is recommended for vitreous involvement [14], or larval laser photocoagulation. Although one review of the literature found that photocoagulation was generally associated with better visual outcomes, the difference was not statistically significant, possibly due to extensive and irreversible damage typically occurring prior to presentation [94]. Successful treatment of panuveitis and neuroretinitis with systemic ivermectin and steroids has also been reported [99]. Dead subretinal larvae may be observed in the absence of signs of active inflammation.

Unusual Bacterial Infections

Delayed-Onset Postoperative Endophthalmitis

Pathogenesis Delayed-onset postoperative endophthalmitis generally results from intraocular penetration by indolent, often commensal bacteria [100], such as *Propionibacterium acnes*, recently renamed *Cutibacterium acnes* [101], *Actinomyces israelii*, or *Corynebacterium* species. Identifying a specific source often is impossible, but generally it is assumed to be due to transincisional, intraoperative, or postoperative entry by bacteria from skin, eyelashes, or contaminated surgical instruments. In this regard, postoperative leaking of corneal wounds may increase risk. It is thought that indolent organisms remain sequestered in macrophages within the lenticular capsule, protected from killing by the host immune system, but still able to produce antigens and other pro-inflammatory mediators [102]. Nd:YAG capsulotomy can incite endophthalmitis by liberating organisms from the capsule into the anterior vitreous.

Clinical Features Typical onset is generally around 9 months postoperatively, but ranges from weeks to years. A high index of suspicion is often required to make the diagnosis. Patients generally exhibit a recurrent, postoperative anterior uveitis that persists more than 6 weeks postoperatively and which may include granulomatous keratic precipitates. Patients may complain of worsening vision or floaters, but conjunctival injection and eye pain are generally mild. Hypopyon and vitritis are variably present. White opacities on the intraocular lens (IOL) and an enlarging plaque on the lenticular capsule are classic signs, but are not always present. Suspicion should be high when low-grade postoperative inflammation is transiently responsive to topical steroids, but repeatedly recurs after appropriate steroid tapering following apparent resolution. Alternative causes of persistent postoperative inflammation should also be considered, including topical steroid noncompliance or rapid tapering, uveitis due to retained lenticular material, uveitis-glaucoma-hyphema (UGH) syndrome, sympathetic ophthalmia, and other unrelated causes of uveitis.

Laboratory Testing Conventional microscopy and aqueous/vitreous culture have poor sensitivity and low diagnostic yield for identification of the causative organism. Vitreous cultures, which have much greater yield (approximately 25%) than those from aqueous humor samples (nearly zero), almost exclusively grow *S. epidermidis* when positive. Nevertheless, if *C. acnes* (*P. acnes*) is suspected, aerobic and anaerobic cultures should be obtained in both solid media and broth and monitored for at least 2 weeks [102]. PCR of intraocular paracentesis specimens has a much higher sensitivity (80%–90%), with vitreous samples possibly providing a higher yield than those from aqueous [103]. However, PCR availability is limited, and the high risk of sample contamination with commensal organisms increases the risk of false-positive results [102]. Surgical IOL explantation and culture may also be beneficial both for diagnosis and treatment. For *C. acnes*, sonication of explanted prostheses has been demonstrated to improve culture sensitivity in spine and breast implants [104], but this technique has not been applied to IOLs.

Management Diagnostic testing may be of limited value and should not delay empiric treatment. *C. acnes* delayed postoperative endophthalmitis is generally treated with intravitreal vancomycin and may also be sensitive to intravitreal penicillin, cefazolin, cefoxitin, and clindamycin. Empiric treatment with intravitreal vancomycin and ceftazidime is reasonable. Oral administration of a later-generation fluoroquinolone with good ocular penetration, such as moxifloxacin, may also be considered. The associated uveitis should be treated with topical or systemic steroids and possibly cycloplegics.

Intravitreal and systemic antibiotics are often insufficient to clear the infection, presumably due to sequestration of organisms in the capsular bag under residual cortex or posterior to the IOL. In these cases, surgical excision of the posterior capsule, any residual cortex, and IOL may be required, typically by a pars plana approach with simultaneous diagnostic vitrectomy. Intraoperative antibiotic irrigation of the IOL is sometimes successful and can prevent the need for IOL exchange.

Cases

Case 1: Toxoplasmosis

A 20-year-old male college student with no past medical history presented after noticing a blind spot just below the center of his right visual field 5 days prior. He had a history of international travel, including to Africa and Asia, and exposure at home to both dogs and cats. He denied any history of tuberculosis. Vision was 20/40 in the right eye and 20/20 in the left eye. There was a 1+ relative afferent pupillary defect in the right eye. Intraocular pressures were normal. Confrontational visual fields showed an inferior defect in the right eye. Examination was notable for 1/2+ anterior chamber cell with stellate keratic precipitates and 3+ anterior vitreous cell in the right eye. The view on fundoscopic exam was hazy, with a whitish peripapillary lesion superiorly and optic disc edema of the right eye (see Fig. 7.1a). Examination of the left eye was entirely normal. No chorioretinal scars were seen in either eye. OCT showed a large chorioretinal elevation with overlying vitritis and associated subretinal fluid extending to nasal fovea (Fig. 7.2).

The patient was treated empirically for both toxoplasmosis chorioretinitis and *Bartonella* neuroretinitis based on his travel history and exposure to cats. An aqueous humor sample was obtained by anterior chamber paracentesis and sent for PCR testing. He received intravitreal clindamycin and oral trimethoprim-sulfamethoxazole (double-

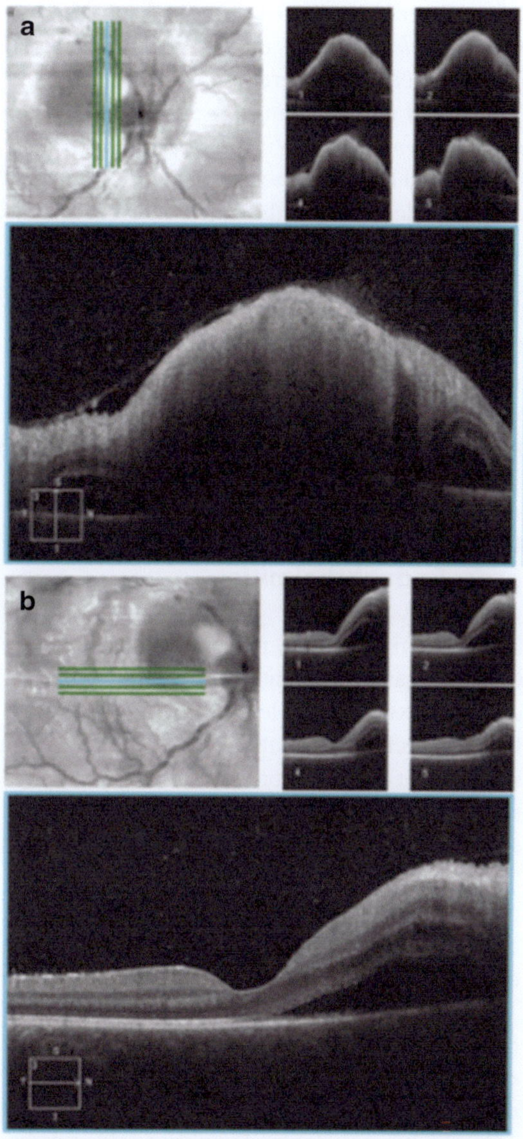

Fig. 7.2 (**a**) OCT scan through the lesion demonstrates retinal elevation and hyperreflectivity, posterior shadowing, and subretinal fluid. (**b**) OCT scan through the macula demonstrates a focal exudative retinal detachment with subretinal fluid extending to the nasal fovea. Images courtesy of Careen Lowder

strength, twice daily) for toxoplasmosis, oral azithromycin for *Bartonella*, and oral prednisone (60 mg daily) for his vitritis. Serum angiotensin-converting enzyme levels (obtained to assess for possible sarcoidosis) were normal, and serologic testing was negative for HIV, syphilis, *Toxocara*, *Bartonella*, and *Toxoplasma* IgM. Tuberculosis testing by interferon-γ release assay was also negative. *Toxoplasma* IgG testing was positive, as was *Toxoplasma* PCR on the aqueous sample. Azithromycin was therefore discontinued after 3 days, and oral clindamycin (300 mg four times per day) was added. Vitritis improved over the next several days, the chorioretinal lesion consolidated and decreased in thickness on OCT, and the subretinal fluid resolved. Nine days after initial presentation, his right eye vision improved to 20/20-3, and his visual field defect resolved. Prednisone was tapered (by halving the dose weekly for 3 weeks) and then stopped. The patient was subsequently followed by his local ophthalmologist and continued to improve.

Case 2: Delayed Postoperative C. *acnes* Endophthalmitis

A man in his early 70s presented approximately 6 months after uneventful, sequential bilateral cataract extraction. He developed iritis and keratic precipitates in the left eye shortly after surgery that improved only minimally on topical steroids (eventually escalated to difluprednate) and oral acyclovir. He denied exposure to TB or STDs and had no other systemic signs of inflammation or infection. An extensive viral, bacterial, and parasitic workup and evaluation for sarcoidosis were negative.

His vision without correction was 20/50 in the right eye and finger counting at 3 feet in the left eye. Pupils and intraocular pressures were normal bilaterally. He had corneal scarring, mild corneal edema, and trace Descemet folds bilaterally. The right eye exam was otherwise unremarkable. In the left eye, there were pigmented keratic precipitates on the inferior corneal endothelium, 1+ anterior chamber cell, and no iris atrophy (Fig. 7.3). A posterior chamber IOL was noted with a hazy posterior capsule without obvious plaque, and there was opacification of the peripheral, anterior capsule with a small accumulation of white material superiorly on the IOL. There was significant vitreous haze and debris and chorioretinal atrophy and scarring. Diagnostic vitreous tap and intravitreal antibiotic injection (vancomycin and ceftazidime) were performed. Cultures grew *C. acnes* within 1 week. He underwent pars plana vitrectomy of the left eye with posterior capsulotomy and vancomycin irrigation of the IOL.

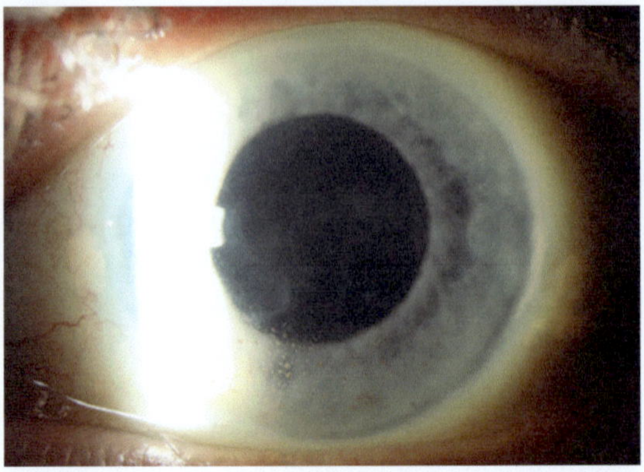

Fig. 7.3 Slit lamp photo demonstrating inferior corneal keratic precipitates and whitish opacities on PCIOL in a patient with postoperative *P. acnes* infection. Image courtesy of Angela Bessette

By 3 months postoperatively, uncorrected vision improved to 20/150 in the left eye. However, his vision worsened to finger counting a month later, with an associated recurrence of anterior uveitis. At this point, he underwent repeat vitrectomy with excision of the remaining lens capsule, IOL explantation, insertion of a scleral-sutured IOL, and intravitreal vancomycin injection. He subsequently did well with improvement in vision to 20/150 by pinhole. His postoperative course was complicated by an epiretinal membrane for which he underwent subsequent membrane peeling.

Case 3: Delayed Postoperative Micrococcus Endophthalmitis

A woman in her mid-70s with a history of Fuchs corneal endothelial dystrophy and diabetes mellitus without retinopathy presented with chronic panuveitis beginning after a complicated right eye cataract surgery 7 months earlier. The intraocular lens implant dislocated posteriorly during this initial procedure and was subsequently repositioned by a pars plana approach. Her inflammation had been unresponsive to aggressive topical steroid therapy. Prior to referral to our clinic, she underwent a basic infectious and uveitic workup, which was unrevealing.

On examination, vision with correction in the right eye was 20/80 and 20/40 in the left eye, which was amblyopic. Intraocular pressures were normal. Corneal guttata were noted bilaterally. The left eye exam was otherwise unremarkable. Examination of the right eye revealed subconjunctival prolene haptics from the 3-piece IOL, located 1 mm posterior to the superior and inferior limbi, with very thin conjunctiva overlying the inferior haptic (Fig. 7.4, **left**). There was 4+ anterior chamber cell, and the inferior edge of the IOL appeared to be tilted anteriorly. On gonioscopy, the inferior haptic was noted to perforate the peripheral iris before exiting the globe (Fig. 7.4, **right**). Posterior exam revealed 3+ vitreous cell, a mild epiretinal membrane, and peripheral endolaser scars.

The differential diagnosis included UGH syndrome due to iris chafing by the anteriorly rotated optic and iris-perforating haptic, as well as chronic exogenous endophthalmitis with ocular entry suspected via prior exposure of the inferior haptic. A vitreous aspiration was performed for culture, and an intravitreal injection of vancomycin and ceftazidime was performed. Topical steroids and cycloplegics were continued. One week later, the vision had improved to 20/70 (pinhole 20/50) in the right eye with 1+ anterior chamber and vitreous cell. Gram stain was negative, but cultures grew pan-sensitive *Micrococcus* species. The patient continued to do well overall, but developed cystoid macular edema consistent with a superimposed UGH syndrome or pseudophakic cystoid macular edema. The patient ultimately underwent repeat IOL exchange with a scleral fixated lens via pars plana approach. Her intraocular inflammation resolved, she was tapered off steroids, and following a subsequent DSAEK, her vision in the right eye was 20/50.

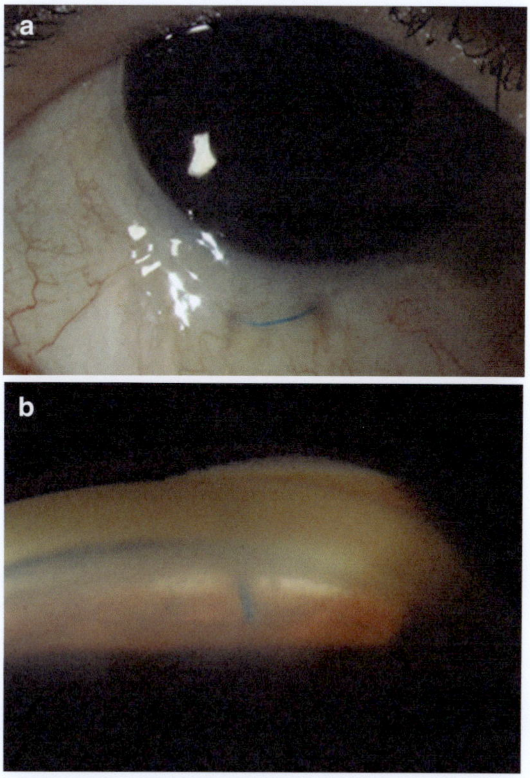

Fig. 7.4 (**a**) Inferior intraocular lens haptic with very thin layer of overlying conjunctiva. (**b**) Goniophotograph demonstrating perforation of inferior peripheral iris by haptic. Images courtesy of Angela Bessette

Compliance with Ethical Requirements The authors declare that they have no conflicts of interest.

References

1. Jones JL, Kruszon-Moran D, Wilson M, McQuillan G, Navin T, McAuley JB. Toxoplasma gondii infection in the United States: seroprevalence and risk factors. Am J Epidemiol. 2001;154(4):357–65.
2. Jeannel D, Niel G, Costagliola D, Danis M, Traore BM, Gentilini M. Epidemiology of toxoplasmosis among pregnant women in the Paris area. Int J Epidemiol. 1988;17(3):595–602.
3. Onadeko MO, Joynson DH, Payne RA. The prevalence of toxoplasma infection among pregnant women in Ibadan, Nigeria. J Trop Med Hyg. 1992;95(2):143–5.
4. Teutsch SM, Juranek DD, Sulzer A, Dubey JP, Sikes RK. Epidemic toxoplasmosis associated with infected cats. N Engl J Med. 1979;300(13):695–9.

5. Morris MI, Fischer SA, Ison MG. Infections transmitted by transplantation. Infect Dis Clin N Am. 2010;24(2):497–514.
6. Guerina NG, Hsu HW, Meissner HC, Maguire JH, Lynfield R, Stechenberg B, et al. Neonatal serologic screening and early treatment for congenital toxoplasma gondii infection. The New England regional toxoplasma working group. N Engl J Med. 1994;330(26):1858–63.
7. Subauste CS, Ajzenberg D, Kijlstra A. Review of the series "disease of the year 2011: toxoplasmosis" pathophysiology of toxoplasmosis. Ocul Immunol Inflamm. 2011;19(5):297–306.
8. Park Y-H, Nam H-W. Clinical features and treatment of ocular toxoplasmosis. Korean J Parasitol. 2013;51(4):393–9.
9. Norose K, Mun H-S, Aosai F, Chen M, Piao L-X, Kobayashi M, et al. IFN-gamma-regulated toxoplasma gondii distribution and load in the murine eye. Invest Ophthalmol Vis Sci. 2003;44(10):4375–81.
10. McCannel CA, Holland GN, Helm CJ, Cornell PJ, Winston JV, Rimmer TG. Causes of uveitis in the general practice of ophthalmology. UCLA Community-based uveitis study group. Am J Ophthalmol. 1996;121(1):35–46.
11. Holland GN. Ocular toxoplasmosis: a global reassessment. Part I: epidemiology and course of disease. Am J Ophthalmol. 2003;136(6):973–88.
12. Pleyer U, Schlüter D, Mänz M. Ocular toxoplasmosis: recent aspects of pathophysiology and clinical implications. ORE. 2014;52(3):116–23.
13. Holland GN. Ocular toxoplasmosis: a global reassessment. Part II: disease manifestations and management. Am J Ophthalmol. 2004;137(1):1–17.
14. Padhi TR, Das S, Sharma S, Rath S, Rath S, Tripathy D, et al. Ocular parasitoses: A comprehensive review. Surv Ophthalmol. 2017;62(2):161–89.
15. Smith JR, Cunningham ET. Atypical presentations of ocular toxoplasmosis. Curr Opin Ophthalmol. 2002;13(6):387–92.
16. Talabani H, Asseraf M, Yera H, Delair E, Ancelle T, Thulliez P, et al. Contributions of immunoblotting, real-time PCR, and the Goldmann-Witmer coefficient to diagnosis of atypical toxoplasmic retinochoroiditis. J Clin Microbiol. 2009;47(7):2131–5.
17. Robert-Gangneux F, Binisti P, Antonetti D, Brezin A, Yera H, Dupouy-Camet J. Usefulness of immunoblotting and Goldmann-Witmer coefficient for biological diagnosis of toxoplasmic retinochoroiditis. Eur J Clin Microbiol Infect Dis. 2004;23(1):34–8.
18. Acers TE. Toxoplasmic retinochoroiditis: a double blind therapeutic study. Arch Ophthalmol. 1964;71:58–62.
19. Soheilian M, Sadoughi M-M, Ghajarnia M, Dehghan MH, Yazdani S, Behboudi H, et al. Prospective randomized trial of trimethoprim/sulfamethoxazole versus pyrimethamine and sulfadiazine in the treatment of ocular toxoplasmosis. Ophthalmology. 2005;112(11):1876–82.
20. Feliciano-Alfonso JE, Vargas-Villanueva A, Marín MA, Triviño L, Carvajal N, Moreno M, et al. Antibiotic treatment for ocular toxoplasmosis: a systematic review and meta-analysis: study protocol. Syst Rev. 2019;8(1):146.
21. Sobrin L, Kump LI, Foster CS. Intravitreal clindamycin for toxoplasmic retinochoroiditis. Retina. 2007;27(7):952–7.
22. Hotez PJ, Wilkins PP. Toxocariasis: America's most common neglected infection of poverty and a helminthiasis of global importance? PLoS Negl Trop Dis. 2009;3(3):e400.
23. Despommier D. Toxocariasis: clinical aspects, epidemiology, medical ecology, and molecular aspects. Clin Microbiol Rev. 2003;16(2):265–72.
24. Sabrosa NA, de Souza EC. Nematode infections of the eye: toxocariasis and diffuse unilateral subacute neuroretinitis. Curr Opin Ophthalmol. 2001;12(6):450–4.
25. Tian JX, O'Hagan S. Toxocara polymerase chain reaction on ocular fluids in bilateral granulomatous chorioretinitis. Int Med Case Rep J. 2015;18(8):107–10.
26. de Graaf P, Göricke S, Rodjan F, Galluzzi P, Maeder P, Castelijns JA, et al. Guidelines for imaging retinoblastoma: imaging principles and MRI standardization. Pediatr Radiol. 2012;42(1):2–14.
27. de Souza EC, Nakashima Y. Diffuse unilateral subacute Neuroretinitis: report of Transvitreal surgical removal of a subretinal nematode. Ophthalmology. 1995;102(8):1183–6.
28. Agarwal MDA. Gass' atlas of macular diseases: 2-volume set - expert consult: online and print. 5th ed. Edinburgh: Saunders; 2012. p. 1378.
29. de Souza EC, Abujamra S, Nakashima Y, Gass JD. Diffuse bilateral subacute neuroretinitis: first patient with documented nematodes in both eyes. Arch Ophthalmol. 1999;117(10):1349–51.
30. Gass JD, Gilbert WR, Guerry RK, Scelfo R. Diffuse unilateral subacute neuroretinitis. Ophthalmology. 1978;85(5):521–45.
31. Relhan N, Pathengay A, Raval V, Nayak S, Choudhury H, Flynn HW. Clinical experience in treatment of diffuse unilateral subretinal neuroretinitis. Clin Ophthalmol. 2015 Sep;28(9):1799–805.
32. Curragh DS, Ramsey A, Christie S, McLoone E. Case report: a case of diffuse unilateral subacute neuroretinitis (DUSN) in a child. BMC Ophthalmol. 2018;18(1):218.
33. Lima BS, Ramezani A, Soheilian M, Rastegarpour A, Roshandel D, Sayanjali S. Successful Management of Diffuse Unilateral Subacute Neuroretinitis with Anthelmintics, and intravitreal triamcinolone followed by laser photocoagulation. J Ophthalmic Vis Res. 2016;11(1):116–9.
34. Natesh S, K H, Nair U, Nair K. Subretinal worm and repeat laser photocoagulation. Middle East Afr J Ophthalmol. 2010;17(2):183–5.

35. Jindal A, Pathengay A. Role of adjunctive laser photocoagulation in a clinical setting of invisible subretinal worm. Can J Ophthalmol. 2013;48(4):e92–3.
36. Gass JD, Callanan DG, Bowman CB. Successful oral therapy for diffuse unilateral subacute neuroretinitis. Trans Am Ophthalmol Soc. 1991;89:97–112. discussion 113–116.
37. Kershaw WE, Lavoipierre MM, Beesley WN. Studies on the intake of microfilariae by their insect vectors, their survival, and their effect on the survival of their vectors. VII. Further observations on the intake of the microfilariae of Dirofilaria immitis by Aedes aegypti in laboratory conditions: the pattern of the intake of a group of flies. Ann Trop Med Parasitol. 1955;49(2):203–11.
38. Gordon RM, Crewe W. The deposition of the infective stage of Loa loa by Chrysops silacea, and the early stages of its migration to the deeper tissues of the mammalian host. Ann Trop Med Parasitol. 1953;47(1):74–85.
39. Duke BO. Studies on loiasis in monkeys. II.--the population dynamics of the microfilariae of Loa in experimentally infected drills (Mandrillus leucophaeus). Ann Trop Med Parasitol. 1960;54:15–31.
40. Boussinesq M, Gardon J. Prevalences of Loa loa microfilaraemia throughout the area endemic for the infection. Ann Trop Med Parasitol. 1997;91(6):573–89.
41. Gobbi F, Buonfrate D, Boussinesq M, Chesnais CB, Pion SD, Silva R, et al. Performance of two serodiagnostic tests for loiasis in a non-endemic area. PLoS Negl Trop Dis. 2020;14(5):e0008187.
42. Churchill DR, Morris C, Fakoya A, Wright SG, Davidson RN. Clinical and laboratory features of patients with loiasis (Loa loa filariasis) in the U.K. J Infect. 1996;33(2):103–9.
43. Loiasis BM. Ann Trop Med Parasitol. 2006;100(8):715–31.
44. Carme B, Mamboueni JP, Copin N, Noireau F. Clinical and biological study of Loa loa filariasis in Congolese. Am J Trop Med Hyg. 1989;41(3):331–7.
45. Klion AD, Massougbodji A, Sadeler BC, Ottesen EA, Nutman TB. Loiasis in endemic and nonendemic populations: immunologically mediated differences in clinical presentation. J Infect Dis. 1991;163(6):1318–25.
46. Hall CL, Stephens L, Peat D, Chiodini PL. Nephrotic syndrome due to loiasis following a tropical adventure holiday: a case report and review of the literature. Clin Nephrol. 2001;56(3):247–50.
47. Bhalla D, Dumas M, Preux P-M. Neurological manifestations of filarial infections. Handb Clin Neurol. 2013;114:235–42.
48. Eballe AO, Epée E, Koki G, Owono D, Mvogo CE, Bella AL. Intraocular live male filarial Loa loa worm. Clin Ophthalmol. 2008;2(4):965–7.
49. Lucot J, Chovet M. Intraocular loaiasis. Apropos of a case. Med Trop (Mars). 1972;32(4):523–5.
50. Osuntokun O, Olurin O. Filarial worm (Loa loa) in the anterior chamber. Report of two cases. Br J Ophthalmol. 1975;59(3):166–7.
51. Barua P, Barua N, Hazarika NK, Das S. Loa loa in the anterior chamber of the eye: a case report. Indian J Med Microbiol. 2005;23(1):59–60.
52. Satyavani M, Rao KN. Live male adult Loaloa in the anterior chamber of the eye--a case report. Indian J Pathol Microbiol. 1993;36(2):154–7.
53. Carme B, Kaya-Gandziami G, Pintart D. Localization of the filaria Loa loa in the anterior chamber of the eye. Apropos of a case. Acta Trop. 1984;41(3):265–9.
54. Hassan S, Isyaku M, Yayo A, Sarkin Fada F, Ihesiulor GU, Iliyasu G. Adult Loa loa filarial worm in the anterior chamber of the eye: a first report from Savanna Belt of northern Nigeria. PLoS Negl Trop Dis. 2016;10(4):e0004436.
55. Rathinam SR, Ashok KA. Ocular manifestations of systemic disease: ocular parasitosis. Curr Opin Ophthalmol. 2010;21(6):478–84.
56. Korten S, Kaifi JT, Büttner DW, Hoerauf A. Transforming growth factor-beta expression by host cells is elicited locally by the filarial nematode Onchocerca volvulus in hyporeactive patients independently from Wolbachia. Microbes Infect. 2010;12(7):555–64.
57. Center for Disease Control Division of Parasitic Diseases and Malaria. Onchocerciasis [Internet]. 2019 [cited 2021 Feb 26]. Available from: https://www.cdc.gov/dpdx/onchocerciasis/index.html
58. Sabrosa NA, Zajdenweber M. Nematode infections of the eye: toxocariasis, onchocerciasis, diffuse unilateral subacute neuroretinitis, and cysticercosis. Ophthalmol Clin N Am. 2002;15(3):351–6.
59. Hall LR, Pearlman E. Pathogenesis of onchocercal keratitis (river blindness). Clin Microbiol Rev. 1999;12(3):445–53.
60. Duke BO, Garner A. Reactions to subconjunctival inoculation of Onchocerca volvulus microfilariae in pre-immunized rabbits. Tropenmed Parasitol. 1975;26(4):435–48.
61. Sakla AA, Donnelly JJ, Lok JB, Khatami M, Rockey JH. Punctate keratitis induced by subconjunctivally injected microfilariae of Onchocerca lienalis. Arch Ophthalmol. 1986;104(6):894–8.
62. Brattig NW. Pathogenesis and host responses in human onchocerciasis: impact of Onchocerca filariae and Wolbachia endobacteria. Microbes Infect. 2004;6(1):113–28.
63. Ottesen EA. Immune responsiveness and the pathogenesis of human onchocerciasis. J Infect Dis. 1995;171(3):659–71.
64. Dadzie KY, Remme J, Rolland A, Thylefors B. Ocular onchocerciasis and intensity of infection in the community. II. West African rainforest foci of the vector Simulium yahense. Trop Med Parasitol. 1989;40(3):348–54.

65. Kanski JJ, Bowling B. Kanski's clinical ophthalmology: a systematic approach. 8th ed. Philadelphia: Saunders Ltd.; 2015. p. 928.
66. Ayong LS, Tume CB, Wembe FE, Simo G, Asonganyi T, Lando G, et al. Development and evaluation of an antigen detection dipstick assay for the diagnosis of human onchocerciasis. Tropical Med Int Health. 2005;10(3):228–33.
67. Shirey RJ, Globisch D, Eubanks LM, Hixon MS, Janda KD. Noninvasive urine biomarker lateral flow immunoassay for monitoring active onchocerciasis. ACS Infect Dis. 2018;4(10):1423–31.
68. Nimir AR, Saliem A, Ibrahim IAA. Ophthalmic parasitosis: a review article. Interdiscip Perspect Infect Dis. 2012;2012:587402.
69. Brunetti E, White AC. Cestode infestations: hydatid disease and cysticercosis. Infect Dis Clin N Am. 2012;26(2):421–35.
70. García HH, Gonzalez AE, Evans CAW, Gilman RH. Cysticercosis working group in Peru. Taenia solium cysticercosis Lancet. 2003;362(9383):547–56.
71. Madan VS, Dhamija RM, Gill HS, Boparai MS, Souza PD, Sanchete PC, et al. Optic nerve cysticercosis: a case report. J Neurol Neurosurg Psychiatry. 1991;54(5):470–1.
72. Dhiman R, Devi S, Duraipandi K, Chandra P, Vanathi M, Tandon R, et al. Cysticercosis of the eye. Int J Ophthalmol. 2017;10(8):1319–24.
73. Wender JD, Rathinam SR, Shaw RE, Cunningham ET. Intraocular cysticercosis: case series and comprehensive review of the literature. Ocul Immunol Inflamm. 2011;19(4):240–5.
74. Mahendradas P, Biswas J, Khetan V. Fibrinous anterior uveitis due to cysticercus cellulosae. Ocul Immunol Inflamm. 2007;15(6):451–4.
75. Chandra A, Singh MK, Singh VP, Rai AK, Chakraborty S, Maurya OPS. A live cysticercosis in anterior chamber leading to glaucoma secondary to pupillary block. J Glaucoma. 2007;16(2):271–3.
76. Ratra D, Phogat C, Singh M, Choudhari NS. Intravitreal cysticercosis presenting as neovascular glaucoma. Indian J Ophthalmol. 2010;58(1):70–3.
77. Lehman B, Leal SM, Procop GW, O'Connell E, Shaik J, Nash TE, et al. Disseminated Metacestode Versteria Species Infection in Woman, Pennsylvania, USA. Emerg Infect Dis J CDC. 2019;25(7) [cited 2019 Sep 30]; Available from: https://wwwnc.cdc.gov/eid/article/25/7/19-0223_article
78. Gulani AC. Sonographic Diagnosis of Orbital Cysticercus Cyst: The "Hanging Drop Sign". J Diagnos Med Sonogr. 1998;14(3):122–4.
79. Raval V, Khetan V. Spectral domain optical coherence tomography features of subretinal Cysticercus cyst. J Ophthalmic Vis Res. 2012;7(4):347–9.
80. Azad S, Takkar B, Roy S, Gangwe AB, Kumar M, Kumar A. Pars Plana vitrectomy with in vivo cyst lysis for intraocular Cysticercosis. Ophthalmic Surg lasers imaging. Retina. 2016;01;47(7):665–9:665.
81. Beri S, Vajpayee RB, Dhingra N, Ghose S. Managing anterior chamber cysticercosis by viscoexpression: a new surgical technique. Arch Ophthalmol. 1994;112(10):1279–80.
82. Das JC, Chaudhuri Z, Bansal RL, Bhomaj S, Sharma P, Chauhan D. Viscoexpression of anterior chamber cysticercus cellulosae. Indian J Ophthalmol. 2002;50(2):133.
83. Kai S, Vanathi M, Vengayil S, Panda A. Viscoexpression of large free floating Cysticercus cyst from the anterior chamber of the eye by double incision technique. Indian J Med Microbiol. 2008;26(3):277–9.
84. Budke CM. WHO/OIE Manual on Echinococcosis in Humans and Animals: A Public Health Problem of Global Concern. In: Eckert J, Gemmell MA, Meslin F-X, Pawlowski ZS, editors. Office International des Epizooties, Paris, 265 pages, ISBN 92–9044-522-X (Euros 40). Veterinary Parasitology. 2002 2;104(4):357.
85. Thompson RC, Lymbery AJ. Echinococcus: biology and strain variation. Int J Parasitol. 1990;20(4):457–70.
86. Wen H, Vuitton L, Tuxun T, Li J, Vuitton DA, Zhang W, et al. Echinococcosis: advances in the 21st century. Clin Microbiol Rev. 2019;32(2):e00075–18.
87. Peregrine AS, Jenkins EJ, Barnes B, Johnson S, Polley L, Barker IK, et al. Alveolar hydatid disease (Echinococcus multilocularis) in the liver of a Canadian dog in British Columbia, a newly endemic region. Can Vet J. 2012;53(8):870–4.
88. Robertson LJ, Troell K, Woolsey ID, Kapel CMO. Fresh fruit, vegetables, and mushrooms as transmission vehicles for Echinococcus multilocularis in Europe: inferences and concerns from sample analysis data from Poland. Parasitol Res. 2016;115(6):2485–8.
89. Eckert J, Deplazes P. Biological, epidemiological, and clinical aspects of echinococcosis, a zoonosis of increasing concern. Clin Microbiol Rev. 2004;17(1):107–35.
90. Grimm F, Maly FE, Lü J, Llano R. Analysis of specific immunoglobulin G subclass antibodies for serological diagnosis of echinococcosis by a standard enzyme-linked immunosorbent assay. Clin Diagn Lab Immunol. 1998;5(5):613–6.
91. Center for Disease Control Division of Parasitic Diseases and Malaria. Echinococcosis [Internet]. 2019 [cited 2021 Feb 26]. Available from: https://www.cdc.gov/dpdx/echinococcosis/index.html
92. Williams DF, Williams GA, Caya JG, Werner RP, Harrison TJ. Intraocular Echinococcus multilocularis. Arch Ophthalmol. 1987;105(8):1106–9.
93. Sinav S, Demirci A, Sinav B, Oge F, Sullu Y, Kandemir B. A primary intraocular hydatid cyst. Acta Ophthalmol. 1991;69(6):802–4.
94. Lagacé-Wiens PRS, Dookeran R, Skinner S, Leicht R, Colwell DD, Galloway TD. Human Ophthalmomyiasis Interna Caused by Hypoderma tarandi, Northern Canada - Volume 14, Number 1—

January 2008 - Emerging Infectious Diseases journal - CDC. [cited 2019 Sep 30]; Available from: https://wwwnc.cdc.gov/eid/article/14/1/07-0163_article
95. Fernandes LF, Pimenta FC, Fernandes FF. First report of human myiasis in Goiás state, Brazil: frequency of different types of myiasis, their various etiological agents, and associated factors. J Parasitol. 2009;95(1):32–8.
96. Francesconi F, Lupi O. Myiasis. Clin Microbiol Rev. 2012;25(1):79–105.
97. Center for Disease Control Division of Parasitic Diseases and Malaria. Myiasis [Internet]. 2021 [cited 2021 Feb 26]. Available from: https://www.cdc.gov/parasites/myiasis/index.html
98. Custis PH, Pakalnis VA, Klintworth GK, Anderson WB, Machemer R. Posterior internal Ophthalmomyiasis: identification of a surgically removed Cuterebra Larva by scanning electron microscopy. Ophthalmology. 1983;90(12):1583–90.
99. Taba KE, Vanchiere JA, Kavanaugh AS, Lusk JD, Smith MB. Successful treatment of ophthalmomyiasis interna posterior with ivermectin. Retin Cases Brief Rep. 2012;6(1):91–4.
100. Funke G, von Graevenitz A, Clarridge JE, Bernard KA. Clinical microbiology of coryneform bacteria. Clin Microbiol Rev. 1997;10(1):125–59.
101. Scholz CFP, Kilian M. The natural history of cutaneous propionibacteria, and reclassification of selected species within the genus Propionibacterium to the proposed novel genera Acidipropionibacterium gen. nov., Cutibacterium gen. nov. and Pseudopropionibacterium gen. nov. Int J Syst Evol Microbiol. 2016;66(11):4422–32.
102. Deramo VA, Ting TD. Treatment of Propionibacterium acnes endophthalmitis. Curr Opin Ophthalmol. 2001;12(3):225–9.
103. Lohmann CP, Linde H-J, Reischl U. Improved detection of microorganisms by polymerase chain reaction in delayed endophthalmitis after cataract surgery11None of the authors have any proprietary interest in any material presented within this article. Ophthalmology. 2000;107(6):1047–51.
104. Portillo ME, Corvec S, Borens O, Trampuz A. Propionibacterium acnes: An Underestimated Pathogen in Implant-Associated Infections. Biomed Res Int [Internet]. 2013 [cited 2019 Sep 28];2013. Available from: https://www.ncbi.nlm.nih.gov/pmc/articles/PMC3838805/

Index

© Springer Nature Switzerland AG 2023
C. Y. Lowder et al. (eds.), *Emerging Ocular Infections*, Essentials in Ophthalmology,
https://doi.org/10.1007/978-3-031-24559-6

MIX
Papier aus verantwortungsvollen Quellen
Paper from responsible sources
FSC® C105338

If you have any concerns about our products,
you can contact us on
ProductSafety@springernature.com

In case Publisher is established outside the EU,
the EU authorized representative is:
Springer Nature Customer Service Center GmbH
Europaplatz 3, 69115 Heidelberg, Germany

Printed by Libri Plureos GmbH
in Hamburg, Germany